Praise for *Look Up*

"An invitation to be self-aware . . . to live joyfully with greater clarity, energy, and purpose."

—Elle Macpherson, founder of Wellco

"Our mission is helping people hear what their body is already telling them. Look Up is the most human guide I've read to doing exactly that—one small daily shift that changes how you feel."

—Doug Sweeny, Chief Marketing Officer, Oura

"Whole-food nutrition and a well-tuned nervous system are two halves of real health. Look Up makes the second half impossible to ignore."

—Charles C. Dubois, president and CEO, Standard Process Inc.

"Literally a GPS for your new diagnosis of Tech Posture Syndrome—insightful, informative, and illuminating. It identifies the global problem and offers an individual action plan."

—Dr. Louis Sportelli, past president, ACA and NCMIC

"As a chiropractor who sees this condition all day, every word is real and true. We must look up if we ever expect to live a life full of health and hope."

—Selina Sigafoose Jackson, DC, FICA, International Chiropractors Association

"Things are looking up for everyone who reads this book. It's an 'aha!' moment from the very first page that solves one of the most prominent health challenges of the modern age. It will be required reading for everyone in my family."

—Del Bigtree, host of The HighWire

"True vitality comes from engagement—with our bodies, our communities, and our purpose. Look Up is an inspiring reminder that as technology advances, our humanity remains our greatest strength."

—Kevin Jackson, DC

"Look Up arrives at exactly the moment we need it. At a time when the physiological costs of our screen-saturated lives are hiding in plain sight—masked as stress, aging, or just "how things are"—this book does something rare: it names the pattern, explains the mechanism, and hands the reader a practical, immediate way out. The 20-Second Lift alone is worth the read, but the deeper gift is the framework—a way of listening to your own body that compounds in value for the rest of your life. Every person with a spine and a screen should read this book."

—Dr. Joel Bohemier

"This book nails the hidden epidemic so many of us see every day in practice: Tech Posture Syndrome. As the creator of PostureScreen, the leading AI powered posture and movement assessment app used by countless thousands of chiropractors and health professionals, we document exactly what the authors describe: Thousands of hours of forward head posture creating sixty pound loads on the cervical spine. The 20-Second Lift is brilliant as a minimum effective dose. Tools like PostureScreen make the invisible visible, so patients and clinicians can actually track real change. This is a must read."

—Joe Ferrantelli, DC

"An eye-opening read and message; and sadly one that most of us can feel and yet aren't fully tuned into. This book is a catalyst for us to make daily changes that lead to more vitality. When you read Maya's story and the reality of the ramifications neurologically to her whole system—its hits you; her story is us all. Important information for all ages to pay attention to and it's an easy read!"

—Lona Cook, DC

"Well written, comprehensive, with simple, easy to implement strategies. I have counseled my community on breath focused meditation and eye exercises for decades to help support their chiropractic adjustments and their neurology. This tool will take it to the next level for them. This book will transform lives."

—Peter Amlinger, DC

"As a chiropractor for the past forty-six years, I've spent my career teaching patients the importance of keeping their heads up to protect the cervical spine and nervous system. This book beautifully reinforces that message and offers a simple yet powerful reminder that the way we hold our heads can have a lasting impact on our health."

—Michael Smatt, DC

"As a pediatric chiropractor, every day I see how posture influences far more than the spine—it shapes breathing, movement, nervous system function, and even a child's ability to learn and thrive. This book has the potential to change the way parents think about human development by helping them understand that looking up isn't just a posture correction—it's a powerful investment in the health and potential of the next generation."

—Dr. Stefanie Gross, chiropractor and founder of Building Brilliant Brains

Look Up

Look Up

The New Science of Vitality in the Age of AI

Dr. Gilles A. LaMarche
Dr. Jeff Langmaid
Dr. Jason A. Deitch

Foreword by Dr. Eric Berg

MAHA
BOOKS

A portion of the proceeds goes to MAHA Action 501(c)4.

MAHA Books may be purchased in bulk at special discounts for sales promotion, corporate gifts, fund-raising, or educational purposes. Special editions can also be created to specifications. For details, contact the Special Sales Department, Skyhorse Publishing, 307 Fifth Avenue, 4th Floor, New York, NY 10016 or info@skyhorsepublishing.com.

MAHA Books is an imprint of Skyhorse Publishing, Inc.®, a Delaware corporation.

Visit our website at www.skyhorsepublishing.com.

Please follow our publisher Tony Lyons on Instagram @tonylyonsisuncertain.

10 9 8 7 6 5 4 3 2 1

Library of Congress Control Number: 2026946206

Cover design by David Ter-Avanesyan

Print ISBN: 978-1-63144-126-4
Ebook ISBN: 978-1-63144-127-1

Printed in the United States of America

For every patient who ever sat across from us and said,
"I don't know why, but something is off."

This book is intended for educational and informational purposes only. It is not a substitute for professional medical advice, diagnosis, or treatment. Always seek the guidance of a qualified healthcare provider before making changes to your health or wellness routine.

A note on patient stories: The individual stories in this book are composite illustrations drawn from clinical experience across three practices spanning more than sixty combined years. Names, identifying details, and specific circumstances have been created to protect privacy. Any resemblance to specific individuals is coincidental. The physiological patterns, symptoms, and outcomes these stories illustrate are real and documented.

Contents

Foreword by Dr. Eric Berg xi

A Note Before We Begin: The Man Who Was Supposed to Be Dead xiii

A Note on the Authors of This Book xix

Introduction: Sixty Pounds xxi

PART I—THE COLLAPSE

Chapter 1: The Silent Collapse: How We Became a Heads-Down Civilization 3

Chapter 2: The Crisis You Can't See: What Tech Posture Syndrome Is Doing to Your Children 13

Chapter 3: The Full Cost: Physical, Cognitive, Emotional, Relational 22

Chapter 4: The Science of Looking Up: Posture, Breath, Vision, and the Nervous System 29

PART II—THE PRACTICE

Chapter 5: The Sensory Diet: What Your Nervous System Is Starving For 39

Chapter 6: The Twenty-Second Lift: The Minimum Effective Dose 46

Chapter 7: The Look Up Day: Morning, Evening, Technology, and Movement 54

Chapter 8: Look Up at Work: The Workplace as a Physiological Environment 62

Chapter 9: Looking Up in Relationships: The Most Personal Cost 69

PART III—THE FUTURE

Chapter 10: Why Healthcare Is Failing: The Missing Piece 77

Chapter 11: The Human Doctor: A New Model of Care 87

Chapter 12: Technology Is Not the Enemy: The Rise of Heads-Up Computing 99

Chapter 13: AI, Augmented Reality, and the Future of Human Vitality: The Feedback Loop That Changes Everything 117

PART IV—THE MOVEMENT

Chapter 14: The Three Intelligences: Universal, Innate, and Artificial 133
Chapter 15: The Compound Life: Small Adjustments, Massive Change 140
Chapter 16: A Future That Looks Up: An Invitation 148

Appendix A: The Thirty-Day Look Up Challenge *163*
Appendix B: For Technology Leaders *165*
Appendix C: A Reading Group Guide *170*
Appendix D: The First Thirty Days *175*
Appendix E: A Note on the Science *179*
Appendix F: For Practitioners *180*
Appendix G: Words We Have Redefined: A Short Glossary *184*
Bibliography *187*
About the Authors *193*
Notes *195*
Index *198*

Foreword

I've spent my entire career looking at one major problem: the massive gap between what the human body is actually designed to do, and what modern life forces it to do. That gap is exactly why I wanted to write this foreword.

Let's be clear about one thing. The science in *Look Up* isn't some new, trendy theory. The connection between your posture and your nervous system has been proven by decades of rock-solid research. We are talking about deep respiratory physiology, the vagus nerve, and autonomic neuroscience. These aren't fringe claims. They're published in peer-reviewed journals and taught in graduate programs. Among experts who study the body-brain connection, this is common knowledge.

What *is* new—and what this book does better than almost anything else out there—is connect that heavy science to the exact way you live your life every single day.

I know plenty of researchers who study the dangers of sitting. I know experts who study how screen time ruins your focus, and others who look at the explosion of anxiety and mental health issues. But almost nobody is connecting the dots between all of them. This book finally connects those lines in a way that actually matters to a normal person trying to survive the modern world.

When I first read this work, one specific stat stopped me in my tracks. It wasn't the fact that looking down puts sixty pounds of extra weight on your cervical spine—though that's alarming enough. It was the **eleven hours**. Eleven hours every single day of forcing your body into a posture that your autonomic nervous system reads as a constant state of stress.

It's not an acute crisis; it's a slow burn. It's a background signal running quietly for eleven hours a day, completely resetting your nervous system to a baseline of chronic stress. That is *not* how the human body was designed to run.

Think about the millions of people who feel "off"—people who are chronically tired, slightly anxious, and just feel like a lesser version of themselves, but can't figure out why. This book gives the most coherent, logical explanation for that mystery I've ever seen. The medical mainstream has completely missed this, and this book correctly identifies exactly why they missed it.

I want to speak directly about the section on children, because this is where the situation becomes urgent. We hear a lot about the adolescent mental health crisis, and everyone is arguing about social media and psychology. But almost nobody is talking about the physical, physiological reality. What happens when you put a developing nervous system into a sustained postural collapse? What happens to a growing brain when its capacity for stress regulation and resilience is warped by hours of staring at a tiny screen? This book asks that question bluntly. I hope the research community wakes up and takes it seriously, because the clock is ticking for these kids.

Now, a word about the solution proposed in these pages. I'm a scientist. My natural instinct, when someone tells me that a "twenty-second fix" can shift your nervous system, is to be skeptical. You should be skeptical too. But if you look at how fast the autonomic nervous system responds to posture and breathing, the data is undeniable. The upper cervical spine is highly sensitive. The vagal response to a long exhale happens within a single breath cycle. Shifting your eyes from a narrow screen to a wide view changes your brain chemistry instantly.

The claim here isn't that twenty seconds cures all your problems. The claim is that twenty seconds, done consistently, changes the upstream inputs that run your nervous system. If you change the input, you change the baseline of a body that has been stuck in the wrong position for years. That claim is scientifically sound. I would defend it anywhere.

Read this book. Put it into practice. And if you are a doctor, a teacher, or a parent, ask yourself: *What if this framework is completely right?* Because the evidence shows that it is.

—Dr. Eric Berg
www.DrBerg.com

A NOTE BEFORE WE BEGIN

The Man Who Was Supposed to Be Dead

The office was on the second floor of a medical building in Sudbury, Ontario. I remember the carpet was gray. I remember there was a plant in the corner that needed water. I remember these things because when someone tells you that you have two years to live, the ordinary objects in the room become very precise. Your brain is trying to hold on to something solid.

The specialist was not unkind. He was precise. He showed me the scans, explained what the pressure numbers meant, used words like "progressive" and "irreversible" and "without surgical intervention."

I was forty-eight years old. I had spent twenty-five years telling patients that the body has an Innate Intelligence that, when properly supported, can heal what medicine cannot. I believed this completely. It was not a marketing line. It was the foundation of my entire professional life.

A Word Before I Tell You What Happened

Some of you are sitting where I sat in 2003—across a desk from a specialist who has just told you that your body is failing, and that the path forward involves a procedure you do not want to undergo. Before I tell you what I did and why, I want to be very clear about what I am not telling you to do.

I am not telling you to decline surgery. I am not telling you to refuse a transplant. I am not telling you that what worked in my case will work in yours, or that any specific diagnosis can be addressed by any specific intervention outside of conventional medicine. The decision I made about my own care was made by a forty-eight-year-old chiropractor with twenty-five years of clinical practice, in full knowledge of the risks, with my eyes wide open about what I was choosing and what I was choosing against. It was an unusual decision for an unusual situation, and the outcome I experienced was not predictable from the path I chose.

If a competent specialist has given you a serious diagnosis and recommended a serious intervention, please consider that recommendation seriously. Get a second medical opinion. Get a third if you need to. Make your decision in partnership with people who know your specific case. The story you are about to read is not a treatment plan. It is the story of how I learned to pay attention to a set of upstream variables in my own body that I had spent twenty-five years recommending to other people without applying to myself. That lesson—about attention, about the inputs your nervous system requires, about the gap between knowing and doing—is what the rest of this book is about. The lesson applies to you regardless of what is on your medical chart. The specific decision I made does not.

With that said, here is what happened.

And now a man in a gray office in Sudbury was telling me that my body was failing. That the only thing left to do was cut it open and replace its parts. I saw four more specialists. They all said the same thing with different degrees of urgency. Surgery. Transplant. Two years. Maybe less. The diagnosis was primary pulmonary hypertension, my pulmonary pressure sitting at a staggering 57 mmHg, accompanied by cardiomegaly—an enlarged heart, measuring 2.5 times normal size. The prognosis was grim: I was given less than twenty-four months to live. The medical alternative—a double lung and heart transplant—might buy me a few more years, but such an approach was entirely outside my paradigm.

So, after much prayer and reflection, I retired from practice on April 14, 2004, preparing for what I thought would be my ultimate transition. I remember whispering to myself, "If this is God's calling for my life, I'm okay." Twenty-five years. More than 750,000 patient visits. I wrote letters to my long-term patients, put an ad in *The Timmins Daily Press*. I hugged my staff. I took my name off the door. And then I went home and did something I had not done since I was a young man: I stopped.

I had been in forward motion my entire adult life. There was always a patient to see, a lecture to give, a book to write, a seminar to prepare. The stopping was harder than I had anticipated. The quiet had weight to it. I sat in my house in Timmins in the early spring, watching the snow melt in the yard, and understood for the first time what it feels like to be waiting for something you cannot name. But God had other plans.

The Morning That Changed Everything

I had always woken early, and retirement had not changed that. I was lying in bed before the light came, and I was not asleep but not quite awake either, in that particular state between the two where the mind sometimes produces things you could not have thought your way to.

A series of powerful thoughts arrived with a clarity that I can only describe as not being mine. It was not a voice. It was more like a fact that had been waiting for me to be still enough to receive it. The first was, quite bluntly, *You're an idiot.* Harsh, yes—but true.

You have been preaching the power of chiropractic and the body's innate ability to heal for twenty-five years. There must be something seriously wrong with your spine and nervous system.

This was on May 15, 2004, thirty-one days after my retirement. For twenty-five years I had preached the message of the body's innate healing power, yet I had failed to truly live it myself. Although I had been checked and adjusted weekly or biweekly by different chiropractic friends, I was not under care as a true practice member. I sat there in the dark for a long time with those thoughts, turning them over and over. Here is what made the thoughts really stop me in my tracks: It was true. I was not practicing what I had spent my life preaching, and the moment I saw that clearly, it stopped me—and I began to pay attention in a new way. That is how learning works: It begins the instant the truth becomes impossible to look away from.

Despite spending my career caring for other people's spines and nervous systems, I had not been a committed patient in anyone's office for more than thirty years. I had been adjusted by colleagues, at conferences, or after breaking bread together, or in addition when something was bothering me. But regular, intentional, sustained chiropractic care—the kind I had recommended to thousands of patients as essential maintenance for a healthy nervous system—I had not given to myself for decades.

The cobbler's children, as they say, have holes in their shoes.

I made an appointment with one of the chiropractors who was now running my former practice, as a new patient—with full consultation, examination, and X-rays. What was revealed shocked me: severe subluxations from C7 to T4, an area directly impacting heart and lung function. These subluxations had caused no musculoskeletal pain but were profoundly interfering with vital communication between my brain and the organs that sustained me.

I began getting adjusted five times a week, without exception. Within three months, my pulmonary pressure dropped to 27 mmHg—normal being 15 mmHG. Within one year, it was normal. Within two years, my cardiomegaly (enlarged heart) had completely resolved. There was, however, residual spinal damage—a plastic deformity at T2 that made me prone to subluxations, spinal displacements affecting neurological function in that area, convincing me that returning to active practice was no longer an option.

I am not telling you this as a miracle. I am telling you this as information. The body has an Innate Intelligence. I spent twenty-five years saying this to other people. When I finally gave my own body what it needed—when I addressed the structural barriers that had been disrupting the neurological signals to my heart and lungs—my body did what bodies do when you stop interfering with their capacity to heal. It healed.

By the fall of 2006, I found myself drawn back to service—this time through education. I began volunteering again at Parker Seminars, which eventually led to a position as vice president at Parker University in Dallas. Then, in 2013, Life University's president, Dr. Guy Riekeman, invited me to join his executive team in Marietta, Georgia. I accepted the opportunity and have served there ever since, currently as vice president of university advancement.

"Go to the Track"

On a serene Sunday morning in July 2022, I awoke to a voice—clear, unmistakable: "Go to the track." I looked around the room. No one was there. I heard it again: "Go to the track."

Curiosity outweighed confusion, so I dressed and drove—not to the nearby high school track, but instinctively to the campus track at Life University, where I have worked since 2013. I walked with purpose, surrounded by birdsong and the whisper of wind through leaves. The experience stirred something long forgotten: the pure joy of running I had known as a young man.

That morning, I decided I would train again, and by summer 2023, I would compete "just one more time." Within weeks, I met Coach Keith Wright, who began preparing me for the masters track and field circuit. In August I shared my vision with my good friend Charlie DuBois, president of Standard Process, a whole-food nutraceutical company based in Palmyra, Wisconsin. He encouraged me to attend his lab in North Carolina. After testing they suggested nutraceuticals that would support my physiology and optimize my performance, and I chose to follow their suggestions.

By December, my coach encouraged me to enter the indoor track competition season—just for experience. That "experience" led to a gold medal in the 400m at the Southeast U.S. Track and Field Association Masters Championship in Norfolk, Virginia, then on to Nationals in Louisville, Kentucky, and finally the World Indoor Championships in Toruń, Poland, all within seven weeks. I was hooked.

During 2023, my first year as a masters athlete, I earned nine gold medals and one silver. In the summer of 2024, I trained alongside a rising star, Macy Tarlton, a former US National Weightlifting Champion and Olympic bobsled hopeful, whose dedication and support elevated my own passion. She was introduced to me by my current coach, Dominic Demeritte, who also coaches the Life University track and field teams. Coach Dominic poured his knowledge, his skill, his inspiration, and his belief into me and prepared me for the 2025 World Championship. My "why" became crystal clear: to demonstrate the power of chiropractic not just to heal but to *elevate human performance*—to win a medal at the 2025 World Championship, twenty years after I was supposed to die. That was my purpose and my vision.

The Finish Line

In 2024, at the World Championships, I suffered a devastating injury—a full-thickness tear of my right rectus femoris and multiple microtears in surrounding muscles. Recovery was long and painful. Yet, on April 8, 2025, six months to the day after my injury, I stepped back onto the track, slow but determined.

In June 2025, I competed at the Southwest Region USATF Masters Championship in Houston, Texas, and won gold in the 400m. It was not an impressive win but I was back competing. By October 2025, I felt ready—this time for the Huntsman World Senior Games World Championship, in St. George, Utah. My first couple races were humbling: fifth in the 200m, sixth in the 800m. Six chances to win a medal, but no medal. Somewhat disappointing. But the next day, I had three more chances—the 400m, my event.

I warmed up carefully, prayed, meditated, and made a simple decision as I was walking up to the start line: *no blocks, standing start, lane 5, vision forward.* The gun fired. I ran with every ounce of life and gratitude in me, with the goal of entering the second curve in line with or ahead of the other competitors. As I entered the final curve, I was in the lead with one other runner, and we were shoulder to shoulder in lanes 5 and 6. And all of a sudden, my heart whispered, or maybe it yelled: "It's time to go."

And I did.

I crossed the line first. A gold medal—and the title of World Champion in the 400m at age seventy—with a time of 1:11.58, a full 1.55 seconds ahead of silver.

Not bad for a man who was told he'd never live past fifty.

Thank God for chiropractic, for its truth, for the power that made the body—and for every soul who has encouraged me on this miraculous journey of grit, commitment, and persistence.

I was supposed to be dead by 2005. I am writing this in 2026. The years I was not supposed to live have been some of the best years of my life. I do not take a single morning for granted.

I still get up before five most mornings to run. No music. I am, as I have always been, the quiet runner who soaks up whatever is around him. Some mornings it is still dark, the air is cold, and the track is empty, and I am seventy-one years old, again standing at the edge of it thinking: Why not?

The answer, every morning, is still the same.

Why I Am Telling You This

Not because I think my situation is comparable to yours. It almost certainly is not. You may not be facing a terminal diagnosis. You are probably not being told you have two years to live.

But here is what I know. The subluxations in my upper spine were not caused by a "rare disease." They were caused by years of accumulated physical stress on a body I had not been tending carefully enough. The principle that correcting them allowed my nervous system to restore the function of my heart and lungs is the same principle at work in every single body that has been spending eleven hours a day looking down at a screen.

The nervous system responds to what you give it. Give it the right inputs—remove the structural barriers, restore the signals, support the Innate Intelligence that is already there—and it does what it was designed to do.

This book is what paying attention looks like.

Why It Matters for What You Are About to Read

The subluxations found in my upper spine—C7 to T4—are precisely in the region most affected by the postural pattern this book is about. The forward head position that screen technology has built into billions of bodies creates mechanical stress on exactly this region, year after year, with consequences that cascade through the nervous system in ways we are only beginning to fully measure.

I was not using a smartphone in 2003. But the spinal dysfunction I carried was the same in kind—if different in cause—as the dysfunction accumulating right now in the bodies of people reading these words.

You do not need to be dying to need what this book offers. You just need to be alive and paying attention.

—Dr. Gilles A. LaMarche
Vice President of University Advancement,
Life University
2025 Gold Medalist in the 400m, Huntsman World Senior
Games World Championships

A Note on the Authors of This Book

We are doctors of chiropractic—three practitioners with more than sixty combined years of clinical experience in a profession that has been built, since 1895, on a clinical tradition centered on the spine, the nervous system, and the body's innate capacity to heal when the structural barriers to that healing are removed. The framework we describe in these pages draws directly on that tradition. We believe—for reasons we will spend much of the book demonstrating—that the convergence of modern neuroscience with the questions our profession has been asking for more than a century puts our field in a unique and timely position to address what we are calling Tech Posture Syndrome at scale.

We have an obvious stake in this argument. We are also among the practitioners who have been thinking about the relationship between spinal function and nervous system state the longest. We trust you to weigh that combination—bias and expertise—and to draw your own conclusions about the case we are making.

We make this disclosure here, at the beginning, because we want you reading the rest of the book with full information about who we are and what we believe. Nothing in the science we cite depends on our profession being right about everything it has historically claimed. Nothing in the practices we recommend—the Twenty-Second Lift, the morning and evening alignments, the threshold practice, the sensory diet—requires you to ever set foot in a chiropractic office. The case for hands-on human care that we will make in chapter 11 is one we believe in deeply, and it is also a case you are entirely free to reject while still benefiting from everything else this book has to offer. We will make the case as well as we can. The conclusion is yours.

This book has three authors and one premise.

Dr. Gilles LaMarche has been a chiropractor for almost fifty years and brings a personal story of physiological restoration that this profession has never had a more powerful voice to tell.

Dr. Jeff Langmaid brings the research synthesis and evidence base that makes every claim defensible to the most rigorous scientific audience.

Dr. Jason Deitch brings two decades of health communication work, a previous book on wellness that anticipated many of these themes before the Heads-Down

World existed, and a personal relationship to the technology story at the center of this argument.

Together, we have written the book that we wished existed when each of us first encountered the patients whose experiences fill these pages—the patients who knew something was wrong but had no name for it, no mechanism, and no path forward. This book is the name, the mechanism, and the path.

The patient stories are composite characters: Maya, Marcus, Daniel, Elena, Sophia, James, and the others are built from real clinical patterns observed across decades of practice. No single person is depicted. The experiences are real. The people are representative. The science is documented in the Notes and Bibliography.

This book was written to be read in order, but any chapter stands alone. If you are a parent, chapter 2 is written for you first. If you are a leader, chapter 8. If you are a clinician, chapters 10 and 11. If you want the science before the protocol, chapter 4. The argument is complete in sequence. The entry points are many.

The individual stories in these pages are composite illustrations drawn from clinical experience spanning more than sixty combined years across three practices, three countries, and tens of thousands of patient encounters. Names, occupations, locations, and identifying details have been created to protect privacy. The physiological patterns, symptoms, diagnostic findings, and outcomes these stories illustrate are real, documented, and consistent with the published research cited in our bibliography.

We chose composite illustrations rather than anonymized real cases for one reason: It allowed us to build characters who embody the full pattern of Tech Posture Syndrome rather than the partial picture any single patient presents. Where individual clinical details might mislead, composite truth clarifies.

Real patient stories—from people willing to be named and identified—will be incorporated in future editions. If you have experienced a transformation through the practices in this book and would like to share your story, please reach out through lookupthebook.com.

One note on Maya, who opens this book and appears across it: She is the most composite of our composite characters—assembled from dozens of people we have known and cared for, the ones whose experience of being slightly less than they used to be, without knowing why, is the reason we wrote this book. If you recognize yourself in her, that recognition is intentional. She is, in the most meaningful sense, all of us.

Now, sit up. Take a full breath. Lift your gaze from the page for just a moment before you turn it.

Then begin.

INTRODUCTION

Sixty Pounds

Maya is thirty-eight years old and she is tired in a way that sleep does not fix.

She knows this tiredness the way you know the furniture in a room you've lived in for years—by feel, in the dark, without having to look. It is there when she wakes up, already present before the alarm, before the first thought of the day. It is there at two in the afternoon when she stares at the second half of a document she has been trying to finish for three days and cannot make herself care about. It is there at dinner when her daughter says something funny and she laughs, genuinely, and then watches the laugh leave her face in the window reflection before her daughter has finished the sentence.

She is not depressed. She has asked herself this question and the answer is no—she still loves her work, still loves her family, still feels joy in the ways she always has. She is just operating at a level that is recognizably below herself. Like a phone that never quite charges to full anymore.

Her doctor has run the tests. Thyroid: normal. Iron: normal. Vitamin D: low, but not dramatically. Sleep study: unremarkable. The blood work comes back clean, and the doctor says what doctors say when the blood work comes back clean: You might want to manage your stress.

Maya is a UX researcher at a technology company. She manages her stress. She goes to yoga on Tuesdays, therapy every other Thursday, takes magnesium at night, and limits herself to one glass of wine. She does everything right. Nothing changes.

What Health Actually Means

There is something else Maya does not know—something that would change not just how she understands her fatigue but how she understands the nature of health itself. She has been taught, as most of us have been taught, that health is the absence of something wrong. You are healthy when the tests come back clean, when the diagnosis is nothing serious, when the specialist says there is nothing to be alarmed about. Health is the state you are in when you are not sick.

This definition is not catastrophic on its face. The results of living by it have been. Not because it is wrong—the absence of disease is genuinely preferable to its presence—but because it is so incomplete as to be functionally useless for the experience Maya is having. Maya is not sick. She is not injured. She has passed every test the healthcare system has designed to detect what is wrong with her. And she feels, unmistakably and persistently, like a fraction of herself.

The definition of health that would help Maya is not the one she was given. It is the one that asks not what is absent, but what is present. Is vitality present? Is the nervous system expressing its full regulatory capacity? Is the body receiving the inputs it requires to maintain the coherence of a living system—the movement, the breath, the sensory variation, the human contact, the structural integrity of the spine that houses the nervous system's primary communication infrastructure? These are not the questions her doctor asked. They are the questions this book asks. And these questions have answers.

The answer in Maya's case is no. Vitality is not fully present, and the reason it is not present is specific, nameable, and reversible. The name for what is happening to her is Tech Posture Syndrome. It is the most widespread condition almost no one has been diagnosed with: a single, nameable enemy hiding inside a thousand vague complaints—the fatigue, the fog, the tight neck, the shallow sleep. Naming it is the first act of defeating it. The mechanism is the sixty-pound number. The reversal begins in twenty seconds.

And the whole of it—the entire practice this book will teach—costs about one minute an hour: twenty seconds, a few times each waking hour, to reset the one system that runs everything else. Less than 2 percent of your day to reclaim the vitality the other 98 percent has been quietly draining. And the fact that neither her doctor nor her therapist nor her yoga instructor have ever said any of this to her is not their failure—it is the failure of a healthcare system that measures the wrong things, organized around a definition of health that was never adequate for the actual experience of being alive.

What no one has asked Maya—not her doctor, not her therapist, not her yoga instructor—is this:

What does your body look like for the ten hours a day you are not exercising or sleeping?

The answer, if Maya could observe herself from outside, would be this: Her head is forward by four to five inches—which translates, based on published biomechanical research, to an effective load of sixty pounds on her cervical spine rather than the ten to twelve pounds it was designed to carry. Her shoulders are rounded. Her chest is slightly collapsed. Her diaphragm has perhaps 60 percent of its normal room to descend. Her breath is shallow. Her visual field is narrow. And her nervous system—reading these physical signals continuously, as it has been doing for seven years—has quietly recalibrated toward a state of low-grade vigilance that feels, from the inside, like vague and inexplicable fatigue.

This is not stress. This is not aging. This is not who Maya is.

This is sixty pounds. Every hour. All day. For seven years.

The number that changes everything is sixty. Not sixty miles, not sixty minutes, not sixty dollars. Sixty pounds—the force your cervical spine bears every hour you spend looking at a screen held at the angle at which you are almost certainly holding it right now.

That number comes from Dr. Kenneth Hansraj, a spinal surgeon who published biomechanical modeling in *Surgical Technology International* in 2014. His finding: A head balanced over the spine exerts approximately ten to twelve pounds of force. Tilt it fifteen degrees forward—the angle of looking at a phone—and that force becomes twenty-seven pounds. Thirty degrees: forty pounds. Forty-five degrees: forty-nine pounds. Sixty degrees, which is the angle most people adopt for sustained reading or scrolling: sixty pounds.

Sixty pounds on a structure designed for twelve. Sustained for three, four, eleven hours a day. Every day. For years.

Before we go further, here is the most important reframe in this book—the one that changes everything that follows:

Your anxiety is not a thought. It is a breath—and you can change it in four seconds. The fatigue is not who you are. It is a posture—and you can begin to change it in twenty seconds. The fog, the low resilience, the half presence at your own dinner table: These are not character flaws or the inevitable cost of modern life. They are physiological states, generated by physical inputs, reversible by different inputs. They are, in significant part, physiological states—strongly influenced by physical inputs and responsive to different ones. This is not a motivational claim. It is a neurological fact. And once you understand it, nothing about your daily experience will look the same.

This book is written for Maya. It is written for the forty-one-year-old software engineer whose headaches started the year he went fully remote. For the executive who has tried every productivity system and still thinks through fog. For the parent who arrives home depleted in a way that feels different from the normal exhaustion of being busy. For the teenager who is anxious in a way that no one around her can explain. For every person who has been told, in effect, that this is just how modern life feels.

A Note on the Science

The scientific framework of this book draws on several established bodies of research, and we want to name them explicitly so that sophisticated readers can evaluate the book on its intellectual foundations.

From neurophysiology and the study of the autonomic nervous system, we draw on the polyvagal framework developed by Dr. Stephen Porges and colleagues across three decades of research—the scientific account of how the vagal system regulates physiological state, social engagement, and the body's capacity for coherent self-organization.

From stress physiology, we draw on the allostatic load framework developed by Dr. Bruce McEwen and colleagues—the scientific account of how the body carries the cumulative cost of sustained stressors and how chronic adaptation produces measurable downstream effects on every major physiological system.

From embodied cognition, we draw on the research of Dr. Amy Cuddy, Dr. Erik Peper, and others who have documented the bidirectional relationship between physical posture and neurological state—the scientific account of how the body shapes the mind as continuously as the mind shapes the body.

From biomechanics, we draw on the cervical loading research of Dr. Kenneth Hansraj and the broader biomechanical literature on forward head posture—the scientific account of what sustained postural demand does to spinal structures and to the nervous system those structures house.

From sensory integration, we draw on the foundational work of Dr. A. Jean Ayres and her successors—the scientific account of how the nervous system processes, integrates, and depends upon specific sensory inputs to maintain regulatory function.

From the literature on compression of morbidity and health span, we draw on the work of Dr. James Fries and others—the scientific account of how the quality of physiological function in later life depends on the quality of physiological investment earlier in life.

Where we cite research in the body of the book, we attempted to represent findings faithfully. Where we extend beyond what any single published study has established—synthesizing across frameworks to describe the pattern we are calling Tech Posture Syndrome—we say so explicitly, and we invite the research community to test the specific claims we are making. The endnotes and bibliography at the back of the book provide the primary-source citations for every empirical claim.

This book is not the first to describe any single piece of what it describes. It is, to our knowledge, the first to integrate these pieces into a unified framework for the specific challenge that modern screen-based life presents to the human nervous system. The integration is our contribution. The science underneath the integration is the shared work of the researchers whose names appear above and whose publications anchor the arguments that follow.

Look Up is also written for Marcus. Marcus is thirty-seven, a VP of product at a technology company, and he has been wearing Meta Ray-Ban Smart Glasses for eight months—not for health reasons, but because they make his mornings more efficient. He takes his first three calls of the day walking. He reads messages through his glasses while he makes coffee. He navigates to meetings without once looking down at a phone. He has not thought about any of this in physiological terms.

He simply noticed, sometime around month three, that he was arriving at his desk in the morning feeling different than he used to. Clearer. More ready. Like the day was already going in the right direction before he sat down. He assumed it was the exercise. It was not only the exercise. This book will tell him what else it was—and why the technology choice he made for convenience reasons was, without his knowing it, one of the best decisions he has made for his nervous system in years.

The Architecture of This Book

Look Up has four organizing ideas. They build on each other. By the end of the book, they will have become a single integrated practice. At the beginning, it helps to see them laid out in order.

The first idea is Tech Posture Syndrome. This is the physical argument—the specific, measurable, reversible pattern that sustained forward head posture is imposing on the bodies of billions of people. It is what this chapter has been describing. It is the problem that makes everything else necessary.

The second idea is PAIN: Pay attention inside now. This is the practice—the discipline of listening to the body's signals rather than suppressing them, of becoming a pain detector rather than a painkiller. PAIN is the practice at the center of this book, and every other practice we teach is an expression of it.

The third idea is adjustment as the operating principle of life. The body adjusts continuously. The mind adjusts continuously. The awareness adjusts by choice. The skilled hands-on care you receive from a human doctor is one expression of the universal activity of adjustment that every living system is already performing. This is the philosophical framework that unifies what you do for yourself (the Twenty-Second Lift), what the body does without your instruction (homeostasis and allostasis), and what a trained clinician does to support both (the Tune-In and Tune-Up).

The fourth idea is the three intelligences—Universal Intelligence, Innate Intelligence, and artificial intelligence. This is the philosophical synthesis. It is the framework that places the current moment—the age of AI—in the larger ordering of human life and that restores the correct priority among the three intelligences operating in every reader's life. The order is the whole argument: Universal Intelligence is the design, Innate Intelligence is that design alive in your body, and artificial intelligence is a tool built to serve the first two—never to replace them.

Trouble begins the moment we invert that order and let the tool we made set the pace for the bodies we were given. Vitality is what becomes possible when we put the order back: human first, body honored, technology in service of life.

All four ideas come together in one integrated practice. One breath. Twenty seconds. A body that is listened to rather than silenced. A life of quality adjustments biased toward vitality rather than depletion. A three-intelligences ordering that keeps the human being—inhabiting a body, paying attention inside now—at the center of the life they are actually living.

That is the architecture. The rest of the book is how it works and what becomes possible when you practice it.

Maya and Marcus are living the same story from opposite ends of it. Maya is experiencing the full cost of the Heads-Down World without knowing why. Marcus is already moving toward the solution without knowing the mechanism. This book meets both of them where they are and gives them what neither currently has: the explanation that makes the experience legible and the practice that makes the direction permanent.

The Pain Paradox: A Little PAIN Now Can Save You a Lot of Pain Later

The single most expensive and destructive misunderstanding in modern health is the cultural consensus that pain is something to be eliminated. This consensus is so pervasive that it is rarely examined. An entire industry is built on it. Billions of dollars a year are spent on it. Hundreds of thousands of lives have been destroyed by opioid addiction built on it. And it is wrong at the most fundamental biological level, because pain is not the problem. Pain is the body's notification system. Eliminating pain without addressing what caused it is the equivalent of disabling the smoke detector because the alarm is annoying.

The body does not begin with pain. The body begins with whispers. A tight neck at the end of a workday. A breath that has gotten shallow. A fog that settles in around three in the afternoon. A sleep that used to be deeper. These are whispers—the body's early-warning system, designed to be heard at a volume that does not disrupt the day. When the whispers are ignored, the body escalates. The whisper becomes an ache. The ache becomes a chronic complaint. The chronic complaint becomes the acute episode that sends a person to the emergency room. The emergency room does what emergency rooms are designed to do: It treats the acute episode with the tools available. The whisper that began the cascade, years earlier, is never discussed, because no one in the emergency room has the time or the framework to discuss it.

The over-the-counter and prescription pain management market in the United States alone generates tens of billions of dollars annually. Opioid pain medications have produced one of the largest public health catastrophes in American history. Every dollar spent on pain suppression is a dollar not spent on pain prevention. Every pill taken to silence a signal is a signal the body will not escalate again in that form; it will escalate in a different form, usually worse, usually later.

The economic argument against the current model of pain management is not controversial. The medical literature on the costs of untreated musculoskeletal dysfunction, opioid dependence, and cascading downstream conditions is extensive. What the literature has not yet named, as a unified cultural phenomenon, is the paradigm that generates all of it: the belief that pain is the enemy rather than the messenger.

From Pain Killer to Pain Detector

Your body is already a pain-detector. It has been operating continuously, reading a dozen signals at once, prioritizing the most urgent, escalating the ones you have not responded to. The question is not whether to install a detection system. The question is whether you are paying attention to the signals the detection system is already sending.

These are two entirely different theories of health.

The painkiller theory says: The symptom is the problem, and the problem should be eliminated.

The pain-detector theory says: The symptom is the information, and the information should be acted upon.

Every healthcare decision a person makes—every pill, every injection, every surgery, every supplement, every lifestyle choice—is made under one theory or the other, whether they know it or not. The population-level adoption of the painkiller theory has produced the population-level health outcomes the United States and most of the Western world is currently experiencing. The population-level adoption of the pain-detector theory would produce different outcomes. Not instantly. Not for everyone. But meaningfully, measurably, and at a scale that would change what healthcare spending, workforce productivity, and daily lived experience look like for hundreds of millions of people.

The practice that makes you a pain-detector rather than a painkiller is already available to you. It has a name. It takes, in its first form, no more than a few seconds. It is the practice this book has been building toward from the moment you began reading. Its name is PAIN.

How This Book Works

The book moves in four stages. Part 1 names the problem and makes it real. Not through statistics alone, but through the specific, lived experience of the people who are in it. Maya, whose diffuse fatigue is the modal experience of the modern knowledge worker. Marcus, whose technology adoption has been inadvertently doing something he did not expect. Daniel, whose posture photograph showed him what five years of remote work had built into his body. Mia, who is nine and whose skull is quietly changing shape. These are composite characters, but the patterns they embody are documented, reproducible, and recognizable.

Part 2 gives you the practice. Not a program with a start date and an end date and a certificate of completion but a set of practices, sized to the minimum effective dose, designed to be attached to what you already do so they require no new time and no exceptional motivation. The Twenty-Second Lift. The sensory diet. The morning and evening alignments. The movement snacks. The threshold practice. These are the specific inputs the nervous system requires, delivered in the format that human behavioral science has consistently found most effective: small, habitual, triggered, compounding.

Part 3 places the practice in its larger context. The healthcare system that did not design for this problem. The Human Doctor (our term for a clinician whose work centers on the body's regulatory capacity rather than waiting for diagnosable breakdown—chapter 11 develops the model in full) model that did. The technology that is beginning to solve the interface problem at civilizational scale. The AI and wearable landscape that will, within a decade, make the practices in this book automatic for anyone who chooses heads-up computing and functional support technology over biometric tracking and pharmaceutical compliance.

Part 4 answers the question that the first three parts of this book make inevitable: If this is true at the individual scale, what does it mean at the civilizational scale? The compound life, the virality of vitality, the society that looks up, the two futures being built simultaneously. And the invitation: not to a program, but to a direction. Upward. Open. Forward. Adapting. Growing. Connected. The direction of a species that spent three hundred thousand years learning to inhabit itself fully—and that is capable of resuming that practice, in twenty seconds, right now.

Before We Go Further

Right now, wherever you are reading this: Notice where your head is. Is it balanced over your spine—ears aligned over shoulders—or has it migrated forward? Notice your shoulders. Notice your breath—when did you last take a breath deep enough to feel your rib cage expand fully?

Now do this:

1. Draw the crown of your head upward, as if a thread attached to the top of your skull is pulling gently toward the ceiling. Feel the cervical spine lengthen.
2. Draw your shoulders back one inch. Let your chest open.
3. Inhale slowly through your nose for four counts—fill your lower lungs first. Hold for a moment. Exhale through your mouth for six to eight counts, fully emptying.
4. Lift your gaze above the horizon. Let your eyes travel to the farthest point available. Let the visual field soften and widen.
5. Make one small movement—a shoulder roll, five steps, a gentle rotation. Break the stillness. Then let a small, genuine smile form—the signal to your nervous system that you are safe, present, and connected.

That is the Twenty-Second Lift. That is the practice at the center of this book.

The shift you just felt is not a trick. It is your nervous system receiving a different set of inputs than it was receiving twenty seconds ago. Your proprioceptive signals have changed. Your vagal tone has begun to shift. Your visual cortex has moved from tunnel mode toward panoramic mode. Your autonomic nervous system has received a signal it is already acting on.

One breath. Twenty seconds.

That is where this begins.

There is one more idea to introduce before we begin, because it frames everything that follows. It is the practice at the center of this book. Every tool we will give you—the Twenty-Second Lift, the morning and evening alignments, the sensory diet, the threshold practice, the Tune-In and Tune-Up—is an expression of a single underlying discipline. The discipline has a four-letter name. The name is designed to make a permanent cognitive change in how you relate to the word it spells: PAIN. Pay attention inside now. A little PAIN now can save you a lot of pain later.

The body communicates in whispers before it screams. A tight neck, persistent fatigue, brain fog, shallow sleep—these are not problems to be suppressed but signals to be read. They are the body saying, in the only language it has, "pay attention inside now." PAIN is the practice of a different response—not silencing the signal but reading it, turning a person from a painkiller into a pain detector.

That is the whole reframe, and the rest of this book will show you how to live it. For now, it is enough to know that the Twenty-Second Lift you just felt is PAIN in physical form, and that this single practice—awareness first, then the lift, the breath, the gaze, the movement—is the discipline at the center of everything that follows.

What becomes possible when you keep going is the subject of everything that follows.

PART I
THE COLLAPSE

How the Heads-Down World Is Dismantling Human Biology

CHAPTER 1

The Silent Collapse

How We Became a Heads-Down Civilization

The most consequential health shift of our era happened one downward glance at a time.

Your body has been trying to tell you something for years.

You just haven't been able to hear it—because you've been looking down.

Not metaphorically. Literally. The average adult in a screen-dependent job now spends approximately eleven hours per day with their head tilted forward and downward, eyes fixed on devices held below eye level. Eleven hours in a position that places sixty pounds of force on a spine designed to carry twelve. Eleven hours of compressed breathing, narrowed vision, and the low-grade nervous system activation that your body interprets—correctly, from a physiological standpoint—as a mild but continuous state of threat.

The neck pain is the least of it.

A Note About Technology

Before we describe what has gone wrong, we want to be specific about what has gone right.

The smartphone is among the most consequential positive inventions in human history. It has placed the accumulated knowledge of the species in the hands of billions of people. It has connected families across continents and given voice to populations that no previous communication infrastructure ever reached. It has transformed access to education, to medicine, to economic opportunity, to community. It has made possible forms of human cooperation at scales that were unthinkable a generation ago. Every author of this book uses these devices every day. We are grateful for them. We believe the future will continue to be shaped by them even more, not less.

The argument we are about to make is not against technology. It is about a specific design completion that the next generation of devices is uniquely positioned to deliver—and about what each of us can do, today, with the tools and the bodies we already have, while that completion is built.

We are not the writers who think the answer to the challenges of the digital era is to use less technology. We are the writers who think the answer is to build better technology, to use it more skillfully, and to develop the physiological literacy that makes the difference between a tool that diminishes us and a tool that extends us. The chapters that follow will name what is going wrong with as much precision as we can. They will also point toward the partners—in the technology industry, in the wearable industry, in healthcare, in workplaces, in the millions of individual readers making millions of individual choices—who are building the way out. The way out exists. It begins with naming what needs to be addressed. Then it gets built.

The Design Decision Nobody Made

In a building in Cupertino, California, sometime in the early 2000s, teams of engineers, designers, and product managers were working on the device that would become the iPhone. They were brilliant people solving genuinely hard problems—how to make a touchscreen responsive at consumer scale, how to fit a usable browser onto a four-inch display, and how to engineer a battery life that would last through a day of use.

They held hundreds of meetings. They ran thousands of tests. They obsessed, with the famous intensity of that "particular company" at that particular moment, over every detail of the user experience.

Not one of those meetings, in any documented record, included a biomechanist.

Not one of those tests measured what happened to the cervical spine of the person holding the device for three hours. Not one of those design reviews asked: At what angle will people naturally hold this? What force does that angle place on the structures of the neck? What happens to those structures if they bear that force for eleven hours a day, 365 days a year, for a decade?

These questions were not asked because they were not within the design frame. The design frame was the screen. The human being holding the screen—their spine, their diaphragm, their autonomic nervous system, their children's developing nervous systems—was outside the frame entirely.

This was not malicious. It was a blind spot. An extraordinarily consequential blind spot, in a product adopted by half the humans on earth.

The engineers who built the first iPhone were not careless people. The documentation from that period—internal memos, design review notes, retrospective accounts from team members who have spoken publicly—reveals a group of extraordinarily talented, intensely motivated, genuinely idealistic people who believed they were building something that would improve human lives. And in many ways, they were right.

The blind spot was not about intent. It was about frame.

The design frame of the early smartphone was the screen. Every decision was evaluated against the question: How do we make this screen more useful, more responsive, more beautiful, more compelling? The question of what the human body does while looking at the screen—the specific angle of the head, the load on the cervical spine, the effect on the diaphragm, the neurological consequences of sustained narrow visual focus—was simply not part of the frame. Not because it was considered and rejected. Because it was never considered.

The Designer's Own Reflection

The designer most closely associated with the iPhone has himself spoken, in public and with characteristic thoughtfulness, about what its design team did and did not fully anticipate. In February 2025, on the BBC's *Desert Island Discs*, Sir Jony Ive—Apple's chief designer through the iPhone era—was asked about his relationship to the device's legacy.

His answer was striking for its candor. Ive acknowledged that while the iPhone produced extraordinary positive contributions—empowerment, connection, liberty for billions of people—the unintended consequences weigh on him. He described innovation as inherently accompanied by unpredicted consequences, said that the unintended nature of those consequences does not diminish his sense of responsibility for them, and explained that this sense of responsibility has shaped decisions he has made since and continues to make. He spoke specifically about the difficulty of using these tools responsibly—acknowledging that even he and his family have had to work deliberately at it—and described the resolve required to not be drawn in and seduced by the very devices he helped design.

We raise this not to criticize Sir Jony Ive. We raise it because his reflection is the acknowledgment that makes the conversation this book is trying to have possible. We are not critics of the smartphone, of the companies that build them, or of their designers. We are observers of the same phenomenon Ive is describing, approaching it from a physiological rather than a cultural angle. The iPhone's cultural consequences—attention, distraction, social connection—have been widely discussed. Its physiological consequences—the sixty-pound load on the cervical spine, the compressed respiration, the attentional narrowing, the cumulative nervous system cost—have not. This book is the physiological chapter of the conversation Sir Jony Ive has himself opened.

This is the defining characteristic of most consequential harm humans have inflicted on themselves through technology: not malice, not negligence in the conventional sense, but a design frame that excludes the question that would have changed everything. What falls outside the frame is invisible—not hidden, not suppressed, just genuinely not seen. And the human body, in the design frame of the digital era, was outside the frame from the beginning.

There is a word for what this kind of incompleteness produces at scale: iatrogenesis—harm caused not by malice but by the unintended consequences of well-intentioned action. Medicine uses it to describe treatments that cause damage the physician did not intend. It applies with equal precision to the smartphone: a device designed to improve human life, which has improved human life in many ways, and which has also produced a specific and measurable pattern of physiological harm that no one intended, in a population of billions, over fifteen years.

Naming it is not an accusation. It is a precondition for addressing it. You cannot fix a problem you have not named. The technology companies that created the problem, if they choose to engage with the science this book documents, have the capacity to accelerate the solution at exactly the scale at which they created the problem. That is the most optimistic possible reading of this moment.

And it was not only Apple. Every smartphone manufacturer, every laptop maker, every monitor designer operated within the same frame. The interface was built for computation. The human biology of the person computing was an afterthought—and in most cases, not even that.

The Heads-Down World was not designed to harm you. It was simply never designed with you—your physical body—in mind. That distinction matters, because it means the harm is not inevitable. It is a design problem. And design problems can be solved.

Meet Maya

Maya, who opened this book, has been using a smartphone since 2012. She got her first laptop for college in 2006. She has worked at a desk, in various forms, for fourteen years. She is, by every external measure, a healthy adult woman in the middle of her life.

What she has never been told—what no one in her healthcare journey has thought to assess—is that her head has spent approximately forty thousand hours in a position that places sixty pounds of force on her cervical spine. That her diaphragm has been operating at roughly 60 percent of its designed capacity for several years. That the anxiety she manages with therapy and magnesium and limited wine has, in significant part, a respiratory dimension that her care has not yet addressed: the predictable neurological consequence of a body that has forgotten how to breathe fully.

The therapy is doing real work. The magnesium helps. The respiratory layer is the piece that has been missing—not a replacement for what she is already doing, but the upstream variable that has been silently amplifying everything she has been trying to manage downstream.

Maya is not a cautionary tale. She is the model human experience of the twenty-first century.

What she is experiencing, as the science shows, is completely reversible.

A Note About the Term "Tech Posture Syndrome"

The cluster of physiological findings we are describing in these pages has not been formally named in the clinical literature. The individual components—forward head posture, upper crossed syndrome, text neck, computer vision syndrome, screen-related musculoskeletal disorders—appear in the research under various labels, none of which captures the full pattern we observe across our patients and across the studies we cite.

We are introducing the term Tech Posture Syndrome deliberately, because naming a pattern is the first step toward addressing it. The pattern is real, the components are documented, and the lived experience of millions of screen-using adults conforms to it with a regularity that warrants a name. Readers and researchers are welcome to disagree with the label. The phenomenon will be there either way.

A Note About the Sixty-Pound Figure

The number comes from a 2014 biomechanical modeling study by Dr. Kenneth Hansraj, published in *Surgical Technology International*, which calculated the cervical load produced by progressive degrees of forward head flexion under static modeling assumptions. The figure represents calculated load at a sixty-degree forward flexion angle. In real-world use, in vivo loading varies considerably based on individual anatomy, the duration of the posture, and the muscular support structures that bear part of the load that the static model assigns to the cervical spine.

The number, in other words, is a useful illustration of the directional relationship—more flexion produces dramatically more cervical load—rather than a precise measurement of what any specific person's spine is bearing in any specific moment. The directional finding it illustrates, that sustained forward head posture meaningfully increases cervical load and produces measurable downstream physiological effects, is robustly supported by the broader biomechanics literature and is the claim the rest of this book builds on.

What Adaptation Actually Means

The human body is the most sophisticated adaptive system on earth. It responds to whatever demands are placed on it with extraordinary precision—and it does not distinguish between adaptations that serve you and adaptations that diminish you. It simply responds to what you repeatedly do.

Hold your head four and a half inches forward for eleven hours a day, and your body will adapt: Anterior muscles will shorten, posterior muscles will lengthen and weaken, joints will stiffen around the position they are held in most often, and the nervous system will recalibrate toward the physiological state that position signals. The body reads collapsed posture as being under load and responds accordingly, maintaining a degree of sympathetic activation appropriate for a threat environment even when no threat exists.

This is not failure. This is the body doing exactly what bodies do. The problem is not the mechanism. The problem is the input. And the input—the postural demand of eleven hours per day in the Heads-Down World—is one that no previous generation of humans has experienced.

Daniel's Photograph

Daniel Ruiz was forty-four, a curriculum developer for an online education platform, working from a home office in Austin, Texas. He had been in that office for five years when he walked into a chiropractic clinic describing himself as "thirty percent less effective than I used to be, with no idea why."

Daniel did not think of himself as someone with a posture problem. He thought of himself as someone with a headache problem, a focus problem, a motivation problem, and an inexplicable tendency to gain weight without changing his diet. He had tried standing desks—he owned two, one for his office and one at his apartment—and found that standing all day made his back hurt in a different location than sitting did. He had tried blue light glasses, productivity timers, and a posture-correcting brace he wore for three days before it began to feel like a punishment. Nothing addressed the "thing" that was happening to his body, because nothing he tried had ever correctly identified what the "thing" was.

The lateral photograph taken by his chiropractor changed this.

His clinician held a phone at shoulder height beside him and showed him the image on the screen. She had placed a plumb line against the wall—a piece of string with a small weight, the simplest tool in clinical measurement—and the line ran straight from ceiling to floor. Daniel's ear that should have lined up over his shoulder was not. It was four and a half inches in front of his shoulder. The equivalent of wearing a forty-nine-pound weight around his neck. All day, every day, for five years.

"That's what I've been carrying?" Daniel asked.

"Yes, that's what you've been carrying."

Daniel was quiet for a moment. Then he said: "And the headaches—"

His doctor replied: "The muscles at the base of your skull. They've been under load for five years trying to hold your head up. By two in the afternoon, they're exhausted. That's your headache."

"And the focus thing?"

"Reduced blood flow to the prefrontal cortex. It's sensitive to postural compression. When your head is forward, the vessels that supply it are slightly compromised—not enough to show up on any scan, but enough to make sustained complex thinking harder than it should be."

Daniel stared at the photograph for a long time. "I thought I was getting old," he said finally. "I thought this was just what forty-four felt like."

It was not what forty-four should feel like. It was what five years of heads-down work in an office with a monitor at the wrong height felt like. It was what Tech Posture Syndrome felt like. And it was reversible.

Six weeks later, his headaches had stopped. Not reduced—stopped. His monitor was at eye level. He had received spinal adjustments three times per week. He had added a fifteen-minute afternoon walk and a five-minute morning mobility sequence. He had not changed his diet, his sleep schedule, his caffeine intake, or anything else. He had changed one thing, the position of his head, and thereby changed the inputs available to his nervous system.

"I feel like I've been driving with the emergency brake on," he said at his six-week check-in, "and someone finally told me how to release it."

That is the most accurate description of Tech Posture Syndrome that any patient has offered in any of our three practices. The emergency brake. On. All day. For years. Not because anything is fundamentally wrong with the car. Because no one ever showed the driver where the brake was, or that it was engaged, and how to release it.

This book is where the brake is, and it tells you how to release it.

"I didn't know I was doing that," Daniel added. "I didn't feel it."

That is the most important sentence in this chapter. He didn't feel it—because it had happened so gradually, one hour of screen work at a time, that his nervous system had recalibrated around it. The collapsed position had become neurologically normal. What he felt instead were the consequences: the headaches, the fatigue, the twelve pounds gained without dietary change, the quality of being present in the room but not quite inside his own life.

The Name for What Is Happening

There is a professional irony embedded in the story of Tech Posture Syndrome that is worth naming directly, because it contains the most important implication for every practitioner reading this book.

The people who most completely understand the mechanism of spinal subluxation, postural adaptation, and nervous system dysregulation—the chiropractors who have spent careers explaining this to their patients—are frequently among the worst examples of their own clinical advice. Not because they do not believe it. Because they are busy. Because "the cobbler's children have holes in their shoes." Because the practitioner who spends eight hours a day supporting other people's spines has often spent zero time supporting their own.

Dr. LaMarche's story, which opens this book, is the most dramatic version of this pattern. A chiropractor who believed completely in the principles of his profession and who, for twenty-five years, did not apply those principles to himself. A twenty-five-year career. The recognition that he had been the cobbler's most barefoot child. The recovery that followed when he finally gave himself what he had been prescribing to others.

The pattern recurs throughout the profession. Survey after survey of chiropractic practitioners finds that a significant proportion do not receive regular chiropractic care themselves, despite recommending it universally to their patients. The reasons are the same reasons that patients give for not practicing the Look Up Practice: no time, no margin, no one to hold them accountable to the practice they know they should have.

This book is addressed to patients. But it is equally addressed to the practitioners who care for them. If you are a chiropractor, a physical therapist, an osteopath, a massage therapist, a health coach—any practitioner whose clinical framework recognizes the nervous system as the primary coordinator of health—this book is asking you the same question it asks every other reader: When did you last give your own nervous system what it needs? Not as a demonstration for patients. As a genuine practice, sustained across months and years, because the compound return applies to your physiology as surely as it applies to theirs.

The practitioner who practices is the practitioner whose patients practice. Modeling is the most powerful clinical intervention available. It requires no technique, no equipment, and no scheduled appointment. It requires only the willingness to apply to yourself what you have been applying to others.

We call it Tech Posture Syndrome.

A Note on the Word Syndrome

We use the word "syndrome" deliberately and precisely. A syndrome, in clinical medicine, describes a cluster of signs and symptoms that consistently appear together and share a common mechanism—without necessarily meeting the criteria for a named disease. Disease implies a discrete pathogen or genetic defect. What we are describing is something more insidious: a pattern. A pattern so normalized that most people experiencing it call it stress, or aging, or just how things are.

Tech Posture Syndrome is the cluster of structural, neurological, respiratory, and cognitive effects that arise from sustained, repetitive interaction with technology in a collapsed physical position. Its mechanism is adaptation. Its cause is environmental. Its solution is not pharmaceutical.

And it is reversible.

Daniel, Six Weeks Later

Six weeks after his posture photograph, Daniel had made three changes: spinal adjustments to restore mobility to joints that had stiffened around his forward head pattern; targeted exercises to reactivate muscles his posture had been suppressing; and one environmental change—he raised his monitor to eye level.

That last one took forty-five minutes and cost nothing.

At six weeks: headaches gone. Sleep improved. The twelve pounds had started to move. He described himself as "twenty percent more present in my own life."

"I didn't realize," he said at his follow-up, "how much energy it takes to be collapsed."

Key Takeaways

- The Heads-Down World was created by a design blind spot, not malicious intent—but the consequences are real and population-scale.
- Tech Posture Syndrome is the predictable physiological result of a body adapting to eleven hours per day of heads-down screen use.
- The body adapts precisely to whatever position it is held in most often, and it does not distinguish between beneficial and harmful adaptations.
- "Syndrome" is the precise term: a cluster of co-occurring conditions sharing a single mechanism, rather than a discrete disease.
- The syndrome develops invisibly, which is exactly what makes it dangerous—its symptoms are felt long before their cause is recognized.

Put It into Practice

Today, ask someone to take one lateral photograph of you in your normal working position. Look at it. Where is your head relative to your shoulders? You do not need to measure anything. You need to see what your body has been doing while you weren't watching. That photograph is the most motivating thing in this chapter—more motivating than any statistic. Please take it and look at it intently before you read chapter 2.

CHAPTER 2

The Crisis You Can't See

What Tech Posture Syndrome Is Doing to Your Children

A generation is growing up with its head tilted forward—
and we are only beginning to count the cost.

In January 2012, the major social media platforms—Facebook, Instagram, Twitter—were in the process of aggressive expansion into mobile. They were building products that would, within eighteen months, be in the pockets of hundreds of millions of adolescents. The engineering teams working on those products were some of the most talented in Silicon Valley. The product managers overseeing them were among the most data-driven in the industry.

Not one of those teams included a child developmental psychologist. Not one of those product reviews incorporated an assessment of what sustained platform use would do to an adolescent's developing attentional system, regulatory capacity, or sense of social identity. The minimum age requirements on these platforms—thirteen, the legal threshold established by the Children's Online Privacy Protection Act of 1998—were widely known to be unenforceable and widely unenforced. Children younger than ten were using these platforms in significant numbers, and no one in any product meeting asked what that meant for a brain that was still forming.

The adolescent mental health data began turning the following year, 2013. The inflection point—the moment when rates of anxiety, depression, self-harm, and suicidal ideation among adolescents began a sustained, multiyear rise across every country that had adopted these platforms—coincides almost exactly with the moment when mobile social media moved from novelty to ubiquity in the hands of young people.

No one in those January 2012 product meetings caused this deliberately. We want to be precise about that. This is not a story about malice. It is a story about a design frame—the same design frame that excluded biomechanists from iPhone development meetings—that did not include the question: What does this do to the children who will use it?

That question was not asked. And its consequences are now visible in fifteen years of adolescent mental health data, in emergency room statistics, in the testimony of an entire generation of young people who grew up inside a system that was never designed with their biology in mind.

And then, six years later, a group of researchers in Australia found something in the bones.

In 2018, researchers at the University of the Sunshine Coast in Australia published a finding so striking it made international headlines—and then disappeared from public conversation with the speed of anything too uncomfortable to sustain.

They had identified bony protrusions forming at the base of the skull in a significant proportion of young adults aged eighteen to thirty. These enthesophytes—growths that form at tendon attachment sites under sustained mechanical stress—had previously been associated almost exclusively with older adults in physically demanding occupations.

The proposed cause: the sustained forward head posture of smartphone use.

These young people's skulls were physically reshaping in response to the postural loads of their device habits.

Read that again slowly: The skulls of young people are changing shape.

What Mia Knows

Mia Chen is nine years old, and she knows things she does not have words for.

She knows, for example, that there are two kinds of times her mother looks at her phone. In the first kind, her mother glances down quickly and comes back—back to the room, back to the conversation, back to her. In the second kind, something different happens. Her mother's face goes somewhere else even though her body stays. Her eyes are on the screen, and her voice is still answering questions, but the answering feels different, like talking to someone through a wall. Mia has never described this. She does not know the phrase "adult attention," or "presence," or "nervous system engagement." She simply knows the difference between the two kinds of looking, and she prefers one of them.

Mia got her first tablet at six—a gift from well-meaning grandparents, loaded with educational apps. She now spends approximately three hours per day on screens, which is below average for her age-group. She is a happy, curious, socially engaged child. By every visible measure, she is thriving.

What no one in Mia's life has measured: the angle of her head during those three daily hours. The postural pattern she is establishing during the years when her nervous system is at its most plastic. The attentional architecture being built in a brain that is spending a significant portion of its waking hours in narrow-focus, close-range, downward-gaze mode.

Mia does not have Tech Posture Syndrome. Not yet. She is nine years old, and her body is resilient, and the accumulation takes time.

But the accumulation has begun.

Mia also knows something about her own body that she has no language for: After an hour on her tablet, something is different. Not bad, exactly. Just different. A kind of flatness that was not there before. A slight heaviness behind her eyes. A sense that the room is less interesting than it was. She usually solves this by asking her mother for a snack, which helps temporarily, and then going back to the tablet, which returns the flatness. She has no reason to connect these two things. She is nine.

But here is what is happening in Mia's body when she sits with her tablet for an hour: Her head is inclined forward by approximately three inches—less than an adult's, because children's devices are often held higher, but still measurably forward. Her diaphragm is partially compressed. Her visual system has been locked in close-range tunnel focus for sixty minutes. Her autonomic nervous system has been running a mild sympathetic activation the entire time—the activation that close-range, high-engagement, reward-cycle digital content reliably produces. The flatness she feels when she puts the tablet down is the nervous system returning, gradually, to its baseline. That baseline is lower than it was an hour ago because it shifts, over time, in the direction of whatever the system is asked to sustain.

Her nervous system is at its most plastic. The patterns being established right now—the attentional architecture, the regulatory baseline, the default relationship between her visual system and the world—are being established during the developmental window most critical for establishing them. And no one in her life has assessed any of this. Not her pediatrician. Not her teacher. Not her mother, who loves her completely and is herself too depleted by her own Tech Posture Syndrome to notice that her daughter's posture has been gradually forward-shifting since age six.

The skull bone study conducted by Australian researchers is real. The enthesophytes are real. Children's skeletons are being physically shaped by the postural demands of device use, in a generation whose parents were told the devices were educational. Both things can be true: The devices contain educational content, and they are reshaping the bodies of the children who use them. The question is whether we will notice before the window closes.

This is what the Heads-Down World is doing to the generation that grew up inside it. Not metaphorically, but structurally.

The Developmental Windows That Cannot Be Reopened

The Windows That Matter Most

Human neurological development does not proceed on a uniform timeline. It proceeds through a series of sensitive periods—windows during which specific neural circuits are preferentially plastic and during which the experiences the developing brain encounters have disproportionate and lasting effects on the architecture of the circuits being built.

The sensitive period for visual processing runs from birth through approximately age eight, with peak plasticity in the first two years of life. The visual system is building its fundamental architecture—the circuits that process depth, motion, spatial relationships, and the integration of near and far focal distance—from the visual inputs it receives. A child who spends the peak visual development years primarily engaging with close-range, two-dimensional, screen-mediated visual environments is building their visual processing architecture around inputs that the system was not designed to receive as a primary diet. The long-term implications for visual processing and attentional architecture are under active investigation and not yet fully characterized. The direction of the evidence is not reassuring.

The sensitive period for attentional regulation runs from approximately age six through twelve, with continuing development through adolescence. The prefrontal systems that coordinate sustained attention, impulse regulation, and the ability to maintain focus in the presence of competing stimuli are being built during exactly the years when children in the developed world are spending increasing proportions of their waking hours with attention-fragmenting digital devices. The attentional architecture a child builds during this window is the attentional architecture they will bring to every academic, professional, and relational challenge for the rest of their life.

The sensitive period for autonomic regulatory capacity—the nervous system's ability to shift between activation states smoothly and return to baseline after challenge—runs from early childhood through late adolescence. The regulatory capacity built during this window is the foundation of emotional resilience, stress management, and the social functioning that depends on the ability to remain physiologically regulated during interpersonal difficulty. A nervous system that builds its regulatory architecture inside an environment of chronic mild sympathetic activation—the environment produced by sustained device use—may be calibrating its baseline and its recovery capacity around inputs that produce lower regulatory resilience than the inputs human nervous systems evolved to receive.

None of these are certain harms. The research is developing and the questions are not fully answered. But the direction is clear enough that waiting for certainty before acting is itself a choice with consequences. The practices in this book are not risky. They are the restoration of inputs the nervous system was designed to receive. The risk is not in practicing them. The risk is in continuing to build children's nervous systems inside an environment of systematic sensory deprivation during the windows when those nervous systems are most plastic and most vulnerable to the shape of the environment they inhabit.

Human neurological development is not linear, and it is not indefinitely plastic. There are specific windows in childhood and adolescence during which neural circuits, cognitive capacities, and regulatory systems are primarily established. What happens during those windows matters in ways that extend across an entire lifetime.

The capacity for sustained attention, developed primarily between ages six and twelve, is shaped by the attentional demands of the child's environment. A child whose primary attentional experience is the fragmented, notification-driven, narrow-focus world of a screen is developing attentional architecture in a fundamentally different context from every generation of children that preceded them.

The regulatory capacity of the nervous system—the ability to manage stress, recover from challenge, and maintain emotional equilibrium—is developed in early childhood through the quality of attachment relationships. But it continues to be shaped throughout adolescence by the physiological environment the developing nervous system inhabits. A chronically dysregulated adolescent—one whose autonomic nervous system has been calibrated by years of postural collapse and attentional narrowing—is developing regulatory capacity under conditions of sustained, low-level physiological stress.

We are not yet certain of all the consequences. But the direction of the evidence is not ambiguous.

The Numbers Nobody Wants to Talk About

Rates of anxiety, depression, self-harm, and suicidal ideation among adolescents—particularly girls—began rising in the United States, the United Kingdom, Canada, and Australia around 2012. The inflection points correlate precisely with the widespread adoption of smartphones among this age-group. The causal debate continues in academic literature. What is not debated is the timing.

What is also not debated—and what is directly relevant to this book—is the physiological dimension of what is happening. An adolescent spending four to six hours per day in the postural and neurological state that the previous chapter described is shaping the physiological baseline from which they experience their emotional life. The baseline from which anxiety is felt. From which social comparison is processed. From which the ordinary challenges of adolescence are navigated.

That baseline, for a significant and growing proportion of young people, is not a healthy one. And it was built one screen hour at a time.

> We are not raising a generation of anxious young people. We are raising a generation of children whose nervous systems have been physiologically dysregulated by an environment that no generation before them has inhabited. The anxiety is a symptom. The Heads-Down World is the cause. The anxiety is, in part, a symptom—and the Heads-Down World is a major and underappreciated contributing factor.

What Parents Can Do—Starting Tonight

The solutions are not simple, and we will not pretend otherwise. Screen use is embedded in the social fabric of adolescent life in ways that cannot be wished away by concerned parents. But some interventions are both achievable and significant:

- **Model before you instruct:** Children learn what normal is by watching the adults in their lives. A parent who practices the Twenty-Second Lift—visibly, at the dinner table, at the doorway, before they answer the phone—is teaching their child what a regulated body looks like. This is more powerful than any rule about screen time.
- **Create screen-free thresholds:** The hour before school. Family meals. The thirty minutes after school before homework. These protected intervals give the developing nervous system regular exposure to what it was designed for: face-to-face contact, open visual environments, physical movement.
- **Teach the vocabulary:** A child who understands, in age-appropriate terms, that looking down for a long time changes how their brain works is a child who has a reason to do something about it. You do not need to teach them biomechanics. You need to teach the connection. "When you look down a lot, your brain gets a little tired. Let's look up for a minute."
- **Advocate at school:** Physical education with a body awareness mandate—postural literacy, breath regulation, movement variety as curriculum—is the highest-return educational investment available. One teacher who understands this and builds two-minute movement breaks into class transitions changes the physiological experience of every child in that room.

A Note About the Skull-Reshaping Research

The 2019 study describing increased prevalence of external occipital protuberances in younger populations—by Shahar and Sayers, published in Scientific Reports[1]—generated significant media attention and subsequent scientific discussion, including methodological critique and questions about the strength of the causal claim. We cite the finding here not as established consensus but as a striking observation that, taken alongside the broader literature on developmental responses to sustained postural demand, points toward a question pediatric and developmental research will need to address with greater urgency in the years ahead.

The deeper claim of this chapter—that childhood and adolescence are developmental windows during which the nervous system is being calibrated by the inputs the environment provides, and that the inputs of the Heads-Down World are categorically different from those of any prior generation—does not depend on this single finding. It rests on the broader literature on developmental neuroscience, on the adolescent mental health data that researchers like Jonathan Haidt have surfaced, and on what every pediatric clinician and every classroom teacher has been observing for the past decade.

The Real Reason This Chapter Is Second

We placed this chapter second—before the science, before the practice, before the workplace and relationship material—because of what we have observed across decades of clinical practice.

Most adults will tolerate a great deal of personal physiological compromise. They will manage the headaches, push through the fatigue, accept the brain fog as the cost of modern productivity. They have been doing it for years and they have built a life around the accommodation.

But show a parent what is happening to their child's skull—to the nervous system that child will inhabit for the rest of their life—and the motivation changes completely.

This book's practices are appropriate for children of almost any age. They require no equipment and take only minutes. They are the most transferable gift in these pages.

Your child is watching what you do with your body. Let what they see be worth learning.

What Ms. Patterson Observed

Keisha Patterson has been teaching fifth grade in a public school in Atlanta for eleven years. She remembers, with the specificity that only teachers develop about their classrooms, the year the tablets arrived.

It was not the year the school introduced them—2019—that she noticed the change. It was the year the pandemic sent children home with their devices for eighteen months, and they came back. That was 2021. She had thirty-two students return to her classroom that fall. She had been teaching fifth grade long enough to know what ten-year-olds looked like. These children looked different.

Their posture, first. She could see it immediately—not in individual children, which would have been unremarkable, but in the whole classroom. When they sat at their desks, the curve of their upper backs was more pronounced than she remembered. Their heads tended forward. When they read, they brought the page toward them rather than sitting toward the page. These were small things in each of them, but taken together, they were the signature of something systemic.

Their attention, second. The attention windows were shorter. Not dramatically, not clinically, but perceptibly. The sustained engagement she had been able to build in her classroom—the thirty-five minutes of deep focus on a long-form text or a complex math problem—now seemed to begin fragmenting around twenty minutes. Not for every child. But for enough children, consistently enough, that she began building her lessons around shorter segments by midyear. Not because pedagogical theory suggested this, but because the children in front of her seemed to need it.

She mentioned this to a colleague, who mentioned it to the school counselor, who said that social media was affecting adolescent attention. Ms. Patterson nodded. But her students were ten. They were not on social media. They had been home on educational tablets, doing the assignments their teachers had sent them, in the position that every child in every home naturally adopts with a device—curled on a couch or floor, head forward, chest collapsed, for hours every day, for eighteen months.

She did not know about the sixty-pound number, the proprioceptive highway, the visual mode, or the vagal tone. She knew what she saw. And what she saw was a classroom of children who had spent a critical developmental period in a specific physical relationship with a specific kind of technology and who had come back changed in ways she could observe but not name.

This book gives her the name. And the name, once known, makes visible what was already there.

Key Takeaways

- Children's skulls are physically reshaping in response to device use—a structural finding that makes concrete what sustained Tech Posture Syndrome does to developing biology.
- Developmental windows in childhood and adolescence make the neurological consequences of the Heads-Down World especially consequential—these effects shape the nervous systems children will inhabit for life.
- The adolescent mental health crisis has a significant, underappreciated physiological component: chronic nervous system dysregulation from years of postural collapse and attentional narrowing.
- Modeling is the most powerful parental intervention: Children learn what normal looks like by watching the adults in their lives.
- This chapter is placed second because protecting a child is often a more powerful motivator than protecting oneself—and the practices in this book serve both.

Put It into Practice

Tonight, before dinner, put all screens face down—including yours—before anyone sits at the table. No announcement. No lecture. Simply create the conditions. Then notice what happens to the quality of conversation, eye contact, and presence in the next thirty minutes. What you observe is what the nervous system was designed for. And it is what you are choosing to protect every time you practice what this book teaches.

CHAPTER 3

The Full Cost

Physical, Cognitive, Emotional, Relational

Tech Posture Syndrome does not stay in the neck.

The Accelerated Aging of the Cervical Spine

Intervertebral disc degeneration may be a normal part of aging. The discs between the cervical vertebrae begin losing hydration and height in the fourth decade of life and continue declining through the fifth and sixth. In a spine that has been loaded normally, this produces mild to moderate changes that most people experience as occasional stiffness and that most clinicians describe as age-appropriate wear.

In a spine that has been loaded with sixty pounds for eleven hours per day for a decade, the picture is categorically different. The accelerated mechanical stress on the anterior disc space—the front of the disc, which bears most of the load in forward head posture—produces degenerative changes at a pace that dramatically outruns the normal aging timeline. Research using MRI comparison of age-matched groups with and without chronic forward head posture consistently finds greater disc degeneration, greater facet joint arthrosis, and greater osteophyte formation in the forward head posture population. The cervical spine of a forty-year-old who has spent fifteen years in sustained forward head posture shows changes more typical of someone fifteen to twenty years older.

These are unlikely reversible findings. The structural changes that accumulate from years of elevated mechanical stress may be permanent. Symptoms can be managed and often managed very well, but the degeneration that produced them is unlikely to be undone. This is the physical argument for early intervention: not that symptoms cannot be addressed later, but that the structural damage being accrued during the years of untreated Tech Posture Syndrome is the kind that compounds, and that preventing the next fifteen years of degeneration from layering on top of the first fifteen is far more consequential than any treatment applied after both have accumulated.

The person who begins addressing their postural pattern at forty-two is not reversing all the degeneration that has accumulated. They are stopping its acceleration. They are giving their cervical spine the chance to age at the pace it was designed to age, rather than the accelerated pace that sustained mechanical overload produces. That is not a small thing. It is the difference between a cervical spine at sixty that functions and one that limits. And it is available, right now, beginning with the position of the head during the eleven hours per day that determine everything.

This is the fact that most people—including most healthcare practitioners who encounter it—fail to fully appreciate: The syndrome begins with a structural pattern, but its consequences extend through every system in the body and every domain of a human life. The neck is where it starts. The rest of a person's experience is where it ends up.

The Accumulation Principle

The costs we have been describing do not exist in isolation. They accumulate. This is the most important single fact about Tech Posture Syndrome and about every other chronic physiological compromise that modern life imposes. The body is an integrated system. It does not experience eleven hours of forward head posture today as a separate event from eleven hours of forward head posture yesterday and eleven hours the day before that. It experiences them as a continuous accumulation.

The scientific framework for this accumulation is called allostatic load. Developed by the neuroscientist Bruce McEwen and colleagues across three decades of research, the allostatic load framework describes how the body carries the cumulative physiological cost of every stressor it encounters—and how chronic adaptation to sustained stress produces measurable, documented changes in nervous system regulation, immune function, cardiovascular health, hormonal balance, and cognitive performance.

Tech Posture Syndrome, in the framework of allostatic load, is not a postural problem. It is a cumulative physiological compromise that began with an unremarkable input—the angle of the head relative to a screen—and has escalated, across years of continuous repetition, into a multisystem pattern that affects how the body heals, how the mind focuses, how the emotions regulate, and how the relationships at the center of a life are actually experienced.

We will return to the allostatic load framework in chapter 11, where we argue that the adjustments a person makes—of awareness, of posture, of clinical care—accumulate in the opposite direction, building what we will call an allostatic reserve. For now, the point to hold is simple. Your body is not keeping separate accounts for each day. It is keeping one cumulative account, across your entire life. Every adjustment you make—and every signal you choose to ignore—is entered into that account. The balance is the quality of the body you will inhabit, at fifty, at sixty, at seventy, at eighty. The math is not mysterious. It is just cumulative.

The Physical Cost: More than Pain

The most immediately obvious cost is structural: Neck pain, tension headaches, shoulder impingement, and upper back dysfunction are now among the most common reasons adults seek medical care in developed countries. A 2019 systematic review in *Applied Ergonomics* found smartphone use significantly associated with neck and shoulder musculoskeletal disorders across multiple populations and study designs.[1]

But the physical cost runs deeper than pain. The sixty-pound load on the cervical spine accelerates degenerative change in intervertebral discs, reduces the mobility of facet joints designed for movement but held in a single position for hours, and creates compensatory tension patterns extending from the base of the skull to the lumbar spine.

Reduced thoracic extension—the ability to open the upper back—impairs shoulder mechanics, increases injury risk, and critically restricts the space available to the diaphragm. The person with Tech Posture Syndrome is not just tight. They are operating with a compressed respiratory system, exchanging a fraction of the air their body was designed to process.

The Cognitive Cost: The Sixty-Pound Strain on the Brain

Research has documented measurable reductions in cerebral blood flow associated with forward head posture. The prefrontal cortex—responsible for complex decision-making, impulse regulation, creativity, and executive function—is exquisitely sensitive to this reduction. The effect is not dramatic enough to notice as "My thinking is worse today." It manifests as "I'm not quite firing on all cylinders"—which is, in fact, exactly what is happening.

There is a second cognitive cost less often measured but perhaps more consequential: attentional narrowing. When the gaze is directed downward and inward toward a screen, the brain's attentional architecture shifts accordingly. The capacity for broad, exploratory thinking—the kind that generates novel solutions, sees unexpected connections, and accesses creativity—is systematically suppressed. People describe this feeling as only being able to think about what is right in front of them. They have not lost the capacity for expansive thinking. They have simply stopped practicing it.

The Emotional Cost: The Body That Generates Mood

A collapsed posture does not merely reflect low energy. It generates it.

This is one of the most important and least-discussed findings in embodied cognition research. The physical position of contraction, sustained over hours, activates physiological processes associated with low mood, reduced motivation, and elevated anxiety—not because of what you are thinking, but because of what your body is doing. The generator, in significant part, is physical. The therapy is addressing the symptom. The body is the cause.

James Okafor was forty-one, a financial analyst at a midsize investment firm in Chicago, when he first described what was happening to him in terms that surprised his clinician: "I'm angry all the time," he said. "Not at anything. Just angry. Like the baseline emotional temperature of my life has gone up by about ten degrees and I can't find the thermostat."

His blood work was clean. His testosterone was in the normal range. He slept adequately. He exercised. He had no clinical reason for the persistent low-grade irritability that had become the ambient emotional weather of his days. His wife had noticed. His children had noticed. He had noticed, which was perhaps the most troubling part—he could see himself being shorter, quicker to frustration, less available to the people who needed him to be available, and he could not explain it and could not stop it.

His posture assessment revealed a forward head position of four inches and significant upper thoracic rounding. His breathing pattern, assessed with a simple hand-on-chest observation, showed predominantly upper-chest breathing with minimal diaphragmatic movement. His respiratory rate at rest was fourteen breaths per minute—within normal range, but at the upper end, and with the shallow volume characteristic of a compressed diaphragm.

His clinician asked him to take three full breaths—really full, rib cage expanding, diaphragm descending, lower belly moving. He sat upright to do it. His eyes changed on the second breath. Something released in his face that he had not known was held.

"I haven't breathed like that in a while," he said.

"When do you think you last did?" his doctor asked.

James thought about it. "I don't know. Maybe not since before COVID. Before we went remote. Before I started working from the couch."

The couch. That was the variable. His office chair had been mediocre but upright. The couch was comfortable in the way that comfortable things are sometimes dangerous—it distributed the load pleasantly, softly, in a configuration that felt restful but placed his diaphragm under exactly the compression his nervous system had been compensating for, for three years, without either of them knowing it.

The anger was not psychological. It was respiratory. A compressed diaphragm, breathing shallowly at the upper end of the normal rate, produces exactly the autonomic profile associated with low-grade irritability: reduced vagal tone, elevated sympathetic baseline, a nervous system running slightly hot. Not enough to be alarming. Enough to change the emotional temperature of a life by ten degrees. Enough to put distance between a man and the people he loves, for reasons none of them can explain.

James's wife told him, eight weeks into his care, that he seemed like himself again. He had not told her what he was doing. She simply noticed that the thermostat had come down.

Maya has been in therapy every other Thursday for two years. Her therapist is skilled and the work is valuable. What the therapy cannot do is change the respiratory mechanics that are producing, through direct physiological pathways, a significant portion of the anxiety she arrives with. That part requires a different intervention.

The Relational Cost: The Collapse That Follows You Home

The collapse that begins at the desk does not stay at the desk. It follows you home—to the dinner table, to the bedroom, to every relationship you are trying to sustain.

A person who has spent eight to ten hours in Tech Posture Syndrome is not, in the moment they look up at their partner or child, physiologically capable of their best relational presence. Their postural system is still oriented toward the screen. Their nervous system is still in its slightly contracted, slightly vigilant mode. The physical signals they are sending—through posture, facial expression, vocal tone—are not the signals of full, open engagement.

Maya knows this feeling. She comes home from work, and she means to be present for Mia, and she is—technically. She is in the room. She is answering questions. She is present enough. But she can feel, in some inarticulate way, that the quality of her presence is not what it should be, that she is giving Mia the performance of attention rather than the thing itself.

The relational cost of Tech Posture Syndrome is the most intimate and the most invisible. It does not show up in medical records. It does not generate a diagnosis. It does not have a treatment code. It shows up in marriages that are technically intact but functionally disconnected, or in parent-child relationships in which the parent is present in the room but absent in the way that children, who are exquisitely sensitive to the quality of attention directed at them, can feel from the other side of the dinner table.

Research in attachment and developmental psychology has documented something that parents who work long hours often discover too late: Children do not primarily evaluate parental love by the quantity of time spent together. They evaluate it by the quality of presence in the time that is shared. A parent who is home for three hours but genuinely present—regulated, open, attentive, eyes not drifting to a device—provides something categorically different from a parent who is home for six hours but physiologically still at the office.

The nervous system does not deceive. A parent who arrives home after ten hours of Tech Posture Syndrome carries, in their body, the postural signature of that accumulation. Their chest is slightly collapsed. Their visual field is still calibrated for eighteen-inch focal distance. Their vagal tone is reduced. Their social engagement circuits—the ventral vagal system that enables the quality of attunement that children need to feel genuinely met—are available but depleted. They will hug their child. They will ask about school. They will sit at the dinner table and participate in the mechanics of a family meal. And something will be missing. The child will feel it. The partner will feel it. And no one will have the language to name what is absent, because the person is there. They are just not fully there.

This is not a character failure. It is a physiological state. And physiological states are changeable—not only through willpower, not only through the decision to be more present, but through the twenty-second practice that changes the physical inputs the nervous system is receiving. Open the chest. Take a full breath. Lift your gaze. The social engagement circuits become available in the ventral vagal state. Creating that state, deliberately, before crossing the threshold into a relationship that deserves it, is the most loving act available to a person who is tired and depleted and trying their best.

Elena, whose story appears in chapter 9, sat in her car for two minutes before going inside so she could be more present walking into her home. Her eight-year-old noticed it within five minutes. This is how fast a child's nervous system reads the quality of a parent's presence. They were built to read it. They read it before any word is spoken. Give them something worth reading.

Key Takeaways

- Tech Posture Syndrome's consequences extend through every system in the body and every domain of life—the neck is where it starts, but the rest of life is where it ends up.
- The physical cost includes structural degeneration, respiratory restriction, and reduced mobility that compounds across years.
- The cognitive cost includes reduced prefrontal blood flow, impaired executive function, and attentional narrowing that systematically suppresses expansive thinking.
- The emotional cost is direct: Sustained physical contraction generates low mood and anxiety through physiological pathway—not psychological cause.
- The relational cost is the most intimate: The collapsed, depleted person who arrives home at the end of the day gives the people they love what is left, rather than what they deserve.

Put It into Practice

Conduct a full-day personal audit. From waking to sleep, track one thing every thirty minutes: your head position. Is it balanced or forward? Your chest—open or collapsed? Your breath—full or shallow? At day's end, tally the hours in each state. The number you find will be the most motivating data point in this book. It will also tell you exactly how much is available to reclaim.

CHAPTER 4

The Science of Looking Up

Posture, Breath, Vision, and the Nervous System

Looking up is not about posture alone.
It is about the nervous system that posture speaks to.

Everything that follows in this book rests on the science in this chapter. The more precisely you understand the mechanism, the more powerfully you will use the practice—and the more readily you will reach for it when the moment of need arrives.

The central claim of this book—the one that makes everything else follow—is this:

Posture is not only a structural issue. It is a neurological one. The position of your body is sending continuous signals to your brain about energy, safety, and capacity. Change the position, and you change the signals. Change the signals, and you change everything downstream.

The Proprioceptive Highway

Your nervous system receives continuous information from your body through proprioception—the sense of position and movement in space generated by specialized receptors throughout the musculoskeletal system. These receptors are densest in the upper cervical spine: the region from the base of the skull to approximately the third vertebra, which functions as something close to a neurological switchboard, sending signals to the brain stem that directly influence breathing rate, heart rate, autonomic balance, and the overall calibration of arousal.

When the head is balanced over the spine—ears over shoulders—these signals tend toward a signature of balance: organized, stable, conducive to what researchers call optimal arousal. The nervous system calibrates accordingly.

Proprioception is the sense that tells you where your body is in space—the position of your limbs, the angle of your joints, the orientation of your head over your spine—without your having to look. It has an inward-facing counterpart: interoception, the sense of the body's internal condition, processed largely through the insula and anterior cingulate cortex. If proprioception reports where you are, interoception reports how you are. The same upper-cervical and vagal pathways that carry postural information also shape this interior sense, which is why a change in posture changes not only how you move but how you feel.

To understand why the Twenty-Second Lift works as quickly as it does—why twenty seconds is genuinely enough to begin shifting neurological state—you need to understand the speed and sensitivity of the proprioceptive system in the upper cervical spine.

The suboccipital muscles—the small, deep muscles at the base of the skull, running from the first and second cervical vertebrae to the occiput—have the highest density of proprioceptive muscle spindles of any muscles in the human body. Per unit of tissue, they carry more positional information to the brain stem than any other structure. This extraordinary density exists because the positional relationship between the head and the spine is among the most critical pieces of information the nervous system receives. Where the head is in space determines where the body is in space, what the eyes can see, and what threats or opportunities the environment contains. The brain stem needs to know this instantly, continuously, and with high precision.

This means two things for the practical purposes of this book. First, the proprioceptive signals from the upper cervical spine reach the brain stem faster than almost any other sensory input—within milliseconds of postural change. Second, because these signals are so informationally dense, even small changes in head position produce immediate and meaningful changes in the data the brain stem is working with. The shift from forward head to neutral position is not a subtle change in proprioceptive terms. It is a significant reorganization of the most sensitive positional sensing system in the body. The brain stem reads it immediately. The autonomic adjustments begin before the conscious mind has registered that anything has changed.

This is why the Lift works in twenty seconds rather than twenty minutes. The mechanism is not slow. The nervous system is not slow. What has been slow is our understanding of how to use it.

Research by Heidi Haavik and colleagues, published in *Neural Plasticity* in 2016, extended this understanding into the realm of neuroimaging.[1] Using functional MRI, Haavik documented that spinal adjustment—the specific clinical intervention that addresses dysfunction in exactly these cervical joints—produces immediate and measurable changes in cortical sensorimotor processing. The brain's map of the body, as visible in fMRI, shifts detectably following adjustment. This is not a structural finding. It is a neurological one. The spine is not merely being moved. The brain is being changed. The map the nervous system uses to coordinate every subsequent action—every movement, every breath, every social gesture—is being updated in real time.

You are not moving bones. You are changing how the brain processes the body's signals. That distinction is the entire argument of this book, stated in the language of neuroimaging.

When the head is displaced forward by four to five inches—as it is during the typical smartphone interaction—the signals from the upper cervical proprioceptors change fundamentally. The brain stem reads a different pattern. And the nervous system adjusts its output. Not dramatically. Subtly. In exactly the way that produces, sustained across years, the constellation Maya experiences as a vague and inexplicable fatigue.

The Breath Connection

The diaphragm requires a specific physical geometry to function at its designed capacity: an upright rib cage, uncompressed anterior chest musculature, and room to descend on inhalation. In the collapsed posture of Tech Posture Syndrome, that geometry is compromised—the diaphragm operates at a fraction of capacity, breathing becomes shallow and driven by the upper chest, and the respiratory rate elevates.

Shallow breathing is not merely inefficient. It is directly dysregulating to the autonomic nervous system. The vagus nerve—the primary pathway between breath and state—is stimulated by slow, deep, extended exhalation. When breath is shallow and rapid, vagal stimulation is reduced. Parasympathetic tone drops. The nervous system drifts toward sympathetic dominance.

The relationship between breath and nervous system state is bidirectional, and understanding both directions is what makes the breath tool kit in chapter 7 so clinically meaningful.

Most people understand that nervous system state affects breathing. When you are anxious, your breathing becomes rapid and shallow. When you are calm, your breathing slows and deepens. This is familiar. The body responds to psychological state with physiological change, including respiratory change. This is well-documented and not contested.

Less commonly understood is that breathing affects nervous system state, through a pathway that bypasses psychological processing entirely. The vagus nerve—the tenth cranial nerve and the primary communication pathway of the parasympathetic nervous system—is stimulated mechanically by the movement of the diaphragm, specifically by the extended exhale. The longer the exhale relative to the inhale, the greater the vagal stimulation, the stronger the parasympathetic signal, the more measurable the shift in autonomic balance toward the rest-and-digest mode.

This means that breath is not merely a reflection of the state of the nervous system. It is an input to the nervous system. And it is an input that you can consciously control in a way that you cannot consciously control heart rate, immune function, or hormonal output. The breath is the only part of the autonomic nervous system with a conscious control override. Every breath practice in the human tradition—from pranayama to the meditation practices of every major contemplative tradition to the physiological sigh documented by Stanford researchers (a double inhale through the nose followed by one long, extended exhale)[2]— is exploiting this override. The traditions discovered it empirically, over thousands of years of practice. Neuroscience has now identified the mechanism.

For the person with Tech Posture Syndrome, the breath dimension is not supplementary to the structural intervention. It is coordinated with it. The collapsed chest prevents the diaphragm from descending. The prevented descent impedes the vagal stimulation. The prevented vagal stimulation reduces parasympathetic tone. The reduced parasympathetic tone elevates the sympathetic baseline. The elevated sympathetic baseline produces the anxiety, the irritability, the shallow resilience, the sense of being slightly on edge in a world that has given you no particular reason to be on edge today.

The structural intervention—the spinal adjustment, the postural correction, the open chest of the Twenty-Second Lift—gives the diaphragm room to move. The breath practice uses that room. Together, they address the respiratory dimension of Tech Posture Syndrome in both directions simultaneously: changing the structure that allows the breath and using the breath to change the nervous system state that the structure had been compromising.

This is the mechanism by which Tech Posture Syndrome generates anxiety in the absence of threat: not through psychology, but through respiratory mechanics. This is one mechanism by which Tech Posture Syndrome can contribute to anxiety in the absence of any real threat: not through psychology alone, but through respiratory mechanics. Maya's therapist is helping her manage the anxiety. But the diaphragm is feeding it.

The Vision Dimension

The Research on Gaze and Cognitive State

The relationship between gaze direction and cognitive mode is one of the more counterintuitive findings in applied neuroscience, and one of the most practically important for the purposes of this book. The intuitive model is that you look down because you are thinking, or focused, or engaged with something demanding. The research suggests the causality also runs in the other direction: Looking down generates a cognitive mode—specifically, the narrow, detail-focused, analytical mode—and looking up or outward generates a different mode—specifically, the broad, associative, creative mode.

Research by Andrew Huberman and colleagues at Stanford has documented the neurological mechanism: The visual cortex's response to panoramic versus narrow gaze involves different activation patterns in the areas of the brain associated with default mode network activity—the network associated with creative thinking, perspective-taking, and the kind of broad associative cognition that generates novel connections between ideas. When the gaze is directed downward and inward at a close-range target, the default mode network is suppressed. When the gaze is directed outward and far, it is activated.

This has a practical implication that most knowledge workers have been intuitively aware of without being able to articulate it: The best ideas rarely come at the desk. They come in the shower, on a walk, looking out a window, in the liminal moment between waking and full alertness. These are moments when the gaze is naturally panoramic or unfocused, when the visual system has left the narrow mode of screen engagement, and when the brain's associative circuitry is activated rather than suppressed.

The knowledge worker who understands this can use it strategically. The hard analytical problem that is not yielding at the desk may yield on a walk, not because the walk provides additional information but because the walk shifts the visual mode, which shifts the cognitive mode, which activates the neural circuits that generate the insight that the analytical mode had been suppressing. The twenty-second Expand element of the Twenty-Second Lift is not a rest from cognitive work. It is a shift to a different kind of cognitive work—the kind that the narrow-gaze mode of sustained screen engagement has been systematically excluding.

For creative professionals, this finding has specific implications. A writing block is often a visual mode problem as much as a content problem. An engineering impasse may be a gaze problem as much as a technical problem. The solution is not to spend more time staring at the screen. It is twenty seconds of looking somewhere else—far, soft, wide—and allowing the neural circuitry that generates the unexpected connection to operate without the suppression that narrow focus imposes.

Where you look influences how you think—not metaphorically, neurologically.

When the gaze is directed downward and inward toward a screen, the visual system enters what neuroscientists call tunnel vision mode. Peripheral awareness is suppressed. The nervous system interprets narrow, close-range visual focus as a signal of potential threat or intense challenge and adjusts arousal accordingly. This is adaptive in the presence of genuine threat. Sustained for eight hours against the backdrop of ordinary desk work, it is the physiological equivalent of running a low-grade alarm all day.

The counterpoint—the panoramic gaze, soft and far-focused—activates the visual system's full range, shifts the nervous system toward parasympathetic activity, and opens the cognitive mode associated with broad, creative, expansive thinking. This is why looking out a window helps, because the visual mode this induces sends a specific neurological signal that the posture and breath have been denying the nervous system all day.

The Convergence of Evidence

What makes this science compelling is not any single study but the convergence across independent research traditions—embodied cognition, respiratory physiology, autonomic neuroscience, and spinal biomechanics—all arriving at the same set of conclusions through different methodological routes.

Heart rate variability (HRV)—the variation in time between heartbeats, now measurable on consumer wearables—has emerged as one of the most robust biomarkers in the research literature, associated with cardiovascular health, immune function, cognitive performance, emotional regulation, and longevity across dozens of independent studies.

Julian Thayer and colleagues' landmark meta-analysis, published in *Neuroscience and Biobehavioral Reviews* in 2012, reviewed 173 studies and concluded that HRV represents a unified index of neurovisceral integration[3]—a direct window into the regulatory capacity of the nervous system. Critically, HRV is measurable in real time, responds to postural and respiratory intervention within minutes, and can be tracked longitudinally on a wrist. The nervous system's health is no longer something that must be inferred. It can be observed directly.

The embodied cognition literature has produced equally striking findings on the behavioral side. A series of studies by Dana Carney, Amy Cuddy, and colleagues at Columbia and Harvard demonstrated that even brief postural interventions—two minutes in an expansive versus constricted body position—produced measurable hormonal changes: increased testosterone and decreased cortisol in the open-posture condition, with opposite effects in the closed-posture condition. (Later replication efforts contested the hormonal findings, though the effects on felt confidence and subjective state have proven more durable.)

Separately, Lisa Feldman Barrett's constructivist model of emotion, developed across decades of neuroscientific research and synthesized in her book, *How Emotions Are Made*,[4] establishes that emotional experience is constructed from interoceptive signals—the body's continuous reporting of its own internal state. The implication is direct: Change the body's state, and you change the emotional experience constructed from it. This is not a metaphor. It is the architecture of how feelings are generated.

This convergence—from biomechanics, from respiratory science, from autonomic neurology, from embodied cognition, from emotion science—is not a fringe claim. It is where the mainstream is going. The practices in this book are not ahead of the science. They are an application of the available science.

A final data point worth noting: The convergence of mind-body and nervous system research is now generating peer-reviewed findings that would have seemed extraordinary a decade ago. A 2025 study published in *Communications Biology*—a journal in the *Nature* portfolio—examined twenty participants before and after a seven-day intensive mind-body retreat combining meditation and reconceptualization practices.[5] Using fMRI, multi-omics, and cellular assays (broad molecular profiling across genes, proteins, and metabolites, paired with cell-level laboratory measures), the researchers documented measurable changes in brain network connectivity and plasma signaling pathways linked to neuroplasticity, metabolism, and neurotransmission. A peer-reviewed EEG study published in a clinical neuroscience journal found significant changes in brain wave patterns in meditation novices after just three days of structured practice. These findings do not validate every claim made in the mind-body wellness space. But they confirm what the broader evidence base has been building toward: Deliberate physical and mental practices produce measurable biological changes, at a speed and depth that the previous scientific consensus did not predict.

The State Chain

These three mechanisms converge in the concept that integrates everything else in this book:

Environment → Posture → Breath → Nervous System State → Behavior → Life Outcomes.

Your environment shapes your posture. Your posture shapes your breath. Your breath shapes your nervous system state. Your nervous system state determines—to a degree most people substantially underestimate—the quality of your thinking, your mood, your resilience, your decisions, and your presence in every relationship you inhabit.

And the chain runs in reverse. Which is the source of everything that follows. Because it means that if you intervene at the level of posture, breath, and gaze—even briefly, even imperfectly—you are intervening at the upstream end of the chain that generates your experience of your own life.

Twenty seconds is enough to move the chain. The practices in this book are the systematic application of that fact, across a day, across a year, across a life.

Key Takeaways:

- Posture is neurological, not merely structural—the upper cervical spine is a primary proprioceptive hub whose signals directly calibrate the autonomic nervous system.
- The collapsed posture of Tech Posture Syndrome mechanically restricts the diaphragm, producing shallow breathing that reduces vagal tone and creates anxiety through a physiological rather than purely psychological pathway.
- Downward visual focus activates tunnel vision mode, which the nervous system interprets as a sustained stress signal.
- The state chain—environment to posture to breath to nervous system state to behavior to outcomes—is the organizing framework of this book, and it runs in reverse.
- Twenty seconds of deliberate intervention at the level of posture, breath, and gaze is enough to begin moving the entire chain—which is why the Twenty-Second Lift works and why it works immediately.

Put It into Practice

The experiment that makes this chapter real: Spend sixty seconds deliberately collapsed—head forward, shoulders rounded, chest caved, breath shallow, gaze downward. Notice your mood, your energy, the quality of your thoughts. Then execute the Twenty-Second Lift from the introduction. Sit fully upright, open the chest, breathe fully, look up, and let the visual field widen. Stay there for sixty seconds. Note what has changed. This is not a demonstration of willpower. It is a demonstration of the state chain in operation. You just ran it in both directions in two minutes.

PART II
THE PRACTICE

The Practices That Reverse the Damage

CHAPTER 5

The Sensory Diet

What Your Nervous System Is Starving For

You feed your body every day. Your nervous system has been going hungry.

We have built an entire culture of nutritional awareness—vitamins, minerals, macronutrients, fiber—around the understanding that the body has specific inputs it requires and that deficiency in those inputs produces specific, predictable dysfunction.

We have not yet applied the same framework to the nervous system.

The nervous system has a diet. Not a metaphorical one—a literal one. Specific sensory and physical inputs that it requires to maintain regulatory function, structural integrity, and the capacity to support the full range of human experience. And modern life, in its current form, is producing a sensory famine—a systematic deprivation of the inputs the nervous system was designed to receive.

> The Look Up Practice is not an exercise program. It is a feeding program. Every practice in the chapters that follow is sensory nutrition—restoring to the nervous system the specific inputs that the Heads-Down World has been denying.

What the Nervous System Requires

Understanding what each of the seven sensory inputs does for the nervous system—not just that it is needed, but why—is what makes the sensory diet framework clinically actionable rather than generically motivating. Each of these inputs was abundant in the environment the nervous system evolved in—bodies that walked, climbed, reached, and rotated; eyes that scanned near and far; faces met in person;

light and sound that varied across the day. Screen-based modern life has quietly stripped nearly all of it away.

1. **Varied movement** provides the proprioceptive variety that the nervous system requires to maintain its spatial map of the body. A body that moves through multiple planes—reaching, rotating, squatting, side-bending—continuously updates the brain stem's model of where the body is in space and what it is capable of. A body that sits still in a single plane for eight hours impoverishes this model, producing the stiffness and coordination degradation that sedentary workers experience because of their work environment rather than recognizing it as a neurological consequence of positional starvation.
2. **Alternating near and far visual focus** maintains the visual system's full functional range. The ciliary muscles that adjust the lens for focal distance, like any muscles, maintain their full range of motion through regular use of that range. Eleven hours of eighteen-inch focal distance produces ciliary muscle fatigue and the progressive loss of near-far flexibility that optometrists are documenting in younger and younger populations. The 20/20/20 principle—every twenty minutes, look twenty feet away for twenty seconds—is not primarily about eye health. It is about maintaining the visual system's full operational range and the attentional benefits of focal variation that the research above describes.
3. **Full respiratory function** maintains the diaphragm's mechanical strength and the vagal stimulation that diaphragmatic movement provides. The diaphragm is a muscle. Like all muscles, it atrophies with disuse and strengthens with use. The compressed diaphragm of sustained seated screen work is not just mechanically inefficient—it is building a pattern of respiratory weakness that compounds across years. The person who has spent a decade breathing primarily from their upper chest has a diaphragm that is functionally weaker than it was, producing a level of respiratory capacity that is below what it would be if the person had been given the input—full diaphragmatic breath, regularly—that maintains it.
4. **Face-to-face social contact** provides the co-regulatory input that the nervous system uses to calibrate its own state in relation to others. Screen-mediated interaction is not a substitute for this. Research comparing in-person and video call interactions finds that the physiological synchronization—the HRV coherence, the micro-expression tracking, the vocal prosody responsiveness—that characterizes in-person engagement is significantly attenuated

in video-mediated interactions, regardless of their emotional content or the participants' intentions.

The social engagement system requires three-dimensional, real-time, physically proximate engagement to operate at full capacity. The remote worker who has been video-calling for three years has been receiving a fraction of the co-regulatory input their nervous system was designed to rely on.

5. **Natural light variation** provides the circadian entrainment signals that regulate the hormonal and neurological rhythms of the body across the day. Melatonin suppression, cortisol rhythm, body temperature cycling, and the timing of the various repair and consolidation processes that occur during sleep are all entrained by the spectrum and intensity of light the person receives across the day. An indoor worker in artificial light is receiving a flattened light spectrum that impairs the precision of circadian entrainment—producing the characteristic sleep disturbance, afternoon energy trough, and difficulty transitioning to wakefulness that knowledge workers frequently report.
6. **Acoustic variety** provides the nervous system with the environmental information it requires to maintain its sense of safety and orientation. Research on soundscapes and autonomic function has found that natural acoustic environments—the varying frequency content, temporal unpredictability, and spatial dimensionality of wind, water, birdsong, and human community activity—produce parasympathetic dominance, while urban noise environments and artificial acoustic monotony tend to maintain sympathetic baseline elevation. The worker in an open-plan office with traffic noise and HVAC hum is receiving an acoustic environment that the nervous system reads as slightly hostile—not dramatically, but enough to contribute to the elevated sympathetic baseline that compounds across the day.
7. **Human touch** activates specific neural pathways—the C-tactile afferents, discovered by researcher Åke Vallbo and colleagues—that are dedicated to the processing of gentle, social touch and that produce oxytocin release, cortisol reduction, and parasympathetic activation through mechanisms entirely distinct from other forms of sensory input. These pathways cannot be activated by any form of digital interaction. They require physical contact. For the single knowledge worker, the person who lives alone or whose primary relationships are conducted remotely, this deficit may be the largest and least-addressed component of their sensory famine.

One further input is worth mentioning, with appropriate caution. Many people report that time spent outdoors in direct contact with the natural world—walking barefoot on grass or sand, sometimes called "grounding" or "earthing"—leaves them calmer and more rested. The research here is genuinely preliminary, drawn from small studies, and the most likely explanation is not any exotic mechanism but the familiar ones already in this chapter: the movement, the natural light, the slower pace, and the reduction in stress that being outside reliably provides. We mention it not as an eighth pillar but as a practical invitation: When you can, take the practice outside. The nervous system that evolved outdoors still responds to being there.

Maya's Sensory Famine

Consider what Maya's body has been signaling, in the language of sensory deficiency, for the past many years.

The tight neck that she has attributed to stress is the proprioceptive system of the upper cervical spine sending an altered signal to her brain stem—not a stress signal, a load signal. The brain stem is receiving information that the head is forward, the load is elevated, and the muscles that maintain that position are in sustained contraction. The brain stem responds as it was designed to respond to that information: by maintaining the level of autonomic activation appropriate for a body under sustained physical challenge. This is not malfunction. It is function, applied to the wrong inputs.

The two o'clock wall she has attributed to poor sleep is the prefrontal cortex running on reduced blood flow after five hours of sustained narrow visual focus and compressed respiratory function. The research on cognitive fatigue is consistent: The kind of fatigue that peaks in the early afternoon in knowledge workers is not primarily about sleep debt. It is about the depletion of the attentional resources that sustained, unvaried close-range screen work consumes without the recovery inputs that would normally replenish them.

A twenty-minute walk at noon—varied movement, alternating visual focus, fresh acoustic environment, full diaphragmatic breath in open air—produces more cognitive recovery than an equivalent period of seated rest. Not because walking is magic. Because it provides, in twenty minutes, several of the sensory inputs the nervous system spent the preceding five hours being denied.

The anxiety she has attributed to the pressures of her job and her life is the autonomic nervous system maintaining a sympathetic baseline that is calibrated to the inputs it has been receiving—not to the genuine threat level of her actual circumstances. Her circumstances are not dangerous. Her physiology has been calibrated as though they were, because the physical inputs she has been providing her nervous system for years are the inputs that signal, at the level of brain stem processing, a mildly threatening environment: collapsed chest, shallow breath, narrow visual field, and sustained stillness. These are the inputs the nervous system reads as early stress indicators. It responds by maintaining a degree of readiness appropriate for an environment generating those signals. The readiness feels, from the inside, like anxiety.

None of these signals are wrong. The nervous system is doing precisely what it was designed to do with the inputs it has been given. The inputs are wrong. And inputs can be changed.

Go through that list with Maya in mind.

Varied movement: Maya works at a desk for nine hours. She goes to yoga on Tuesdays. On the four other workdays, her primary movement is the twenty steps between her desk and the kitchen.

Visual variation: Maya's workday is spent within eighteen inches of two monitors. When she looks away from them, she looks at her phone.

Full respiratory function: Maya's diaphragm, in her typical working posture, is operating at roughly 60 percent capacity. She has not taken a full breath, without conscious effort, in years.

Social contact: Maya works remotely. She has video calls. She sees her colleagues' faces in small rectangles on a screen. She has not been in a room with most of them since 2021.

Natural light: Maya's home office has one window. She rarely opens the blind because the glare hits her screen.

Human touch: Maya is a single parent. The most consistent physical contact in her daily life is Mia climbing into bed with her on Saturday mornings.

This is not a description of a deprived life. This is a description of a normal, successful, modern professional life. And it is a sensory famine.

The fatigue Maya experiences is not mysterious when seen through this lens. It is the predictable neurological consequence of a system being asked to regulate itself without the inputs it requires to do so.

The Reframe That Changes Everything

Understanding the sensory diet changes the emotional relationship to the practices in this book. They stop being things you should do—items on a wellness checklist that generate guilt when skipped. They become things your nervous system needs. The difference in motivation is enormous.

You do not feel guilty about eating when you are hungry. You eat. Hunger is information, and you respond to it.

The fatigue, the brain fog, the anxiety, the shallow resilience—these are data points of information too. They are the nervous system's way of signaling that the diet is deficient. The practices in the chapters that follow are how you respond.

The Science Behind the Sensory Famine

The sensory diet concept is not a metaphor. It is a literal description of how the nervous system maintains its regulatory capacity, grounded in decades of research from occupational therapy, developmental neuroscience, and autonomic physiology.

A. Jean Ayres, the occupational therapist whose sensory integration theory transformed developmental practice in the mid-twentieth century, established that the nervous system processes and organizes sensory information from the body and environment to produce adaptive behavioral responses.[1] When that sensory input is insufficient, variable, or poorly integrated, the regulatory architecture the nervous system uses to manage emotion, attention, and behavior degrades. Ayres worked primarily with children with developmental differences. The framework she established applies with equal precision to typically developing adults whose environment has been systematically stripped of sensory variety.

What the modern knowledge worker's environment produces is a specific pattern of sensory deprivation: high cognitive load paired with low sensory variety, sustained narrow visual focus, minimal proprioceptive input from whole-body movement, reduced acoustic complexity, and dramatically reduced face-to-face social engagement. This is not a neutral environment. It is an environment that systematically starves the nervous system of the inputs it requires to maintain regulatory function—while simultaneously demanding that the nervous system perform its highest-level cognitive operations.

The result is predictable: dysregulation. Not the dramatic dysregulation of a clinical disorder, but the low-grade, persistent dysregulation of a system that is being asked to do complex work without adequate resources. The fatigue, the irritability, the attentional fragmentation, the shallow emotional resilience—these are not symptoms of a disease. They are the adaptive responses of a nervous system that is hungry.

You would not ask a person to run a marathon on an empty stomach and then wonder why they are not performing at their best. You are asking your nervous system to coordinate your entire cognitive, emotional, and relational life on a sensory diet that would not sustain the simplest biological requirements of the system. The hunger is real. The meal is available. It begins with a single full breath.

Key Takeaways

- The nervous system has a sensory diet—specific physical and sensory inputs it requires to maintain regulatory function—and modern life is producing a systematic famine of those inputs.
- The seven inputs most depleted by modern screen-based life: varied movement, visual alternation, full respiratory function, face-to-face social contact, natural light, acoustic variety, and human touch.
- Tech Posture Syndrome is, at its root, the predictable neurological consequence of prolonged sensory deprivation.
- Reframing the Look Up Practice as sensory nutrition rather than exercise or wellness ritual changes the motivational relationship to it—needs are more reliably met than should-dos.
- The fatigue, fog, and anxiety of Tech Posture Syndrome are information: the nervous system signaling that its diet is deficient. The practices in this book are the response.

A Note on Bodies

The protocol described in this book assumes a typical adult body capable of upright sitting, full diaphragmatic breathing, and the small movements described in the Twenty-Second Lift. We are aware that not every reader inhabits that body. Adaptations of every element of this protocol exist for readers with mobility limitations, structural conditions of the spine, respiratory conditions, sensory differences, and a wide range of other circumstances that make the practice as written inaccessible. Readers in these circumstances are encouraged to work with a practitioner familiar with their specific situation—a physical therapist, an occupational therapist, an adaptive movement specialist, or a chiropractor with experience in adaptive care—to translate the principles of the protocol into the practice that fits their body. The principles are universal. The specific movements are not. The benefit of the practice is available to every nervous system that can receive any version of these inputs in any form.

Put It into Practice

Audit your sensory diet using the seven-item list in this chapter. For each input, rate your typical daily provision on a scale of one to ten. The lowest numbers are your highest-priority interventions—the places where your nervous system is hungriest. Begin there. Not with the most impressive practice. With the most urgent deficiency. That is where the largest gain lives.

CHAPTER 6

The Twenty-Second Lift

The Minimum Effective Dose

It takes twenty seconds. It changes the system that runs everything else.

Medical research has a concept called the minimum effective dose: the smallest intervention that produces the desired physiological effect. Below the threshold, nothing meaningful happens. At or above it, the effect is reliable and real.

The Twenty-Second Lift is the minimum effective dose for state change.

You have already practiced it. This chapter will explain precisely why it works, how to make it permanent, and how to extend it into the full Look Up Ritual for moments when you have more than twenty seconds to give.

Why Twenty Seconds Is Enough

The neurological effects of postural change begin within seconds—because the proprioceptive signals from the upper cervical spine reach the brain stem rapidly, and the brain stem's autonomic adjustments begin before the conscious mind has registered that anything has changed.

Research on postural intervention consistently shows that the transition from collapsed to expanded produces detectable autonomic shifts within one to three breath cycles. Mood, self-rated energy, and cognitive clarity show measurable effects within sixty seconds of sustained postural change. Heart rate variability—the most reliable single measure of nervous system regulatory capacity—begins shifting within the first full extended exhale.

The nervous system is extraordinarily responsive to the inputs it receives because it evolved in an environment where physiological states needed to change rapidly. The transition from threat to safety, or from rest to action, needed to happen in moments. That responsiveness, which served our ancestors in acute situations, is available to us in ordinary ones. We simply need to know how to use it.

The Neuroscience of Rapid State Change

The skeptic's question is reasonable: How can twenty seconds change anything meaningful? The answer requires understanding what "meaningful" means at the neurological level, and it turns out to mean something quite different from what the skeptic is imagining.

The skeptic is imagining something meaningful as producing a lasting structural change in the nervous system, rewiring neural pathways, establishing new habits or building long-term regulatory capacity. These things take time. The skeptic is right that twenty seconds does not accomplish them.

But meaningful, in the neurological sense, that matters for the Twenty-Second Lift is more immediate: changing the autonomic state that the nervous system is currently operating from. Not rewiring it. Shifting it. The way you shift a thermostat by adjusting the current setting—without changing the thermostat's fundamental architecture, without rewiring the house, in twenty seconds.

The autonomic nervous system operates through continuous feedback loops. The sympathetic and parasympathetic branches are not fixed states but dynamic balances, updated moment by moment based on the sensory inputs the brain stem is receiving. Change the inputs, and the balance shifts. The question is how quickly.

The answer, based on the convergent evidence in autonomic research, is: faster than you think. Heart rate variability—the most sensitive real-time measure of autonomic balance—begins changing within a single breath cycle when the breath is deliberately extended. The first extended exhale shifts vagal tone. The first shift in vagal tone changes the ratio of sympathetic to parasympathetic activity. The first change in that ratio alters the processing of the prefrontal cortex, which is exquisitely sensitive to autonomic state. The subjective experience of that sequence—the sense of something releasing, something settling, something becoming more possible—arrives within twenty seconds because the mechanism works within twenty seconds.

This is the minimum effective dose in the most precise possible sense. Not the smallest dose that produces any effect. The smallest dose that produces the effect that matters: a shift in the neurological state from which everything else the person does in the next twenty minutes will proceed.

Research by Paul Lehrer, Richard Gervitz, and colleagues has documented that the autonomic effects of brief slow-paced breathing persist for minutes after the practice ends—the system maintains a degree of the shift, rather than snapping immediately back to baseline.[1] This explains why a Twenty-Second Lift at the beginning of a difficult meeting changes the quality of thinking in that meeting. The shift is not confined to the twenty-second time frame. It creates a window. The length of the window depends on what happens next—which is why practicing the Lift at regular intervals, attached to triggers, matters more than any single practice.

The Seven Elements

The Twenty-Second Lift is the physical embodiment of PAIN. It begins with the practice of awareness—one beat of paying attention inside now—and then moves through five physical elements that change the body's state while the awareness tracks what is happening. The awareness is not separate from the physical practice. It is what makes physical practice a practice rather than a mechanical exercise.

The full structure is seven elements: the practice of PAIN first, the five physical movements that flow from it, and a closing practice of PAIN that completes the loop. Counted simply, that is seven things, in order: (1) the practice of PAIN, (2) Lift, (3) Open, (4) Breathe, (5) Expand, (6) Move, and (7) a closing practice of PAIN, sealed with a gentle smile.

PAIN. Pay attention inside now. Before you adjust your posture, adjust your awareness. Two seconds. Notice where your head is. Notice what your breath is doing. Notice the state of your nervous system right now, before you change anything. This inward attention has a name in neuroscience: interoception—the brain's sense of the body's own internal state: the felt sense of your breath, your heartbeat, your muscular tension, your level of activation. Where proprioception tells you where your body is, interoception tells you how it is. Elite athletes spend years on proprioceptive training—drilling balance, joint position, and body awareness until their physical control becomes precise and automatic. The practice of PAIN is the interoceptive equivalent: a deliberate, repeated training of your inward sense, so that reading and regulating your own nervous system becomes just as precise, just as automatic. It is how an ordinary person builds, over time, the internal awareness that lets them perform at their own best—the way a top performer does. And here is the part that makes this practice yours and no one else's. As you train interoceptive perception—day after day, beat after beat—you are building something proprietary: a precise, personal, internal read on what your particular nervous system needs to come back to its best state. Think of it as developing your own internal intellectual property—an IP that belongs to you alone, because no one else has lived in your body, learned its signals, or knows its unique appetite for the inputs that regulate it. PAIN is, in the most literal scientific terms, the deliberate training of that internal intelligence. But the goal is not merely to notice how you feel right now. The deeper aspiration is to listen to your body and compare what you feel against what you know you are capable of feeling—your innate vital capacity.

That comparison is what creates the gap: the honest distance between where your nervous system is today and where it could be with healthy inputs delivered consistently. A clear, hopeful picture of that possible state is not optional. It is the thing that makes the gap worth closing.[2]

This is the tune-in. It is what makes the physical elements that follow a response to something specific, rather than a generic ritual. It is also the practice that, across dozens of daily repetitions, builds the physiological self-literacy that is the long-term goal of everything else in this book.

Then the five physical elements.

Why the Sequence Matters

The seven elements of the Twenty-Second Lift are not interchangeable. They are sequenced to compound each other's neurological effect, each creating the physiological conditions for the next to be more effective than it would be in isolation.

> **Lift** first, before breath, because the structural repositioning of the cervical spine changes the proprioceptive signal the brain stem receives before anything else changes. The brain stem's first information about the shift comes from the upper cervical joints—the most sensitive proprioceptive sensors in the body. When the crown of the head lifts and the cervical spine lengthens, the signal changes immediately. The brain stem begins adjusting its autonomic output before the breath has completed a single cycle.
>
> **Open** second, before the full breath, because the diaphragm cannot descend fully in a collapsed chest. The sequence of postural correction before respiratory engagement is not arbitrary—it is anatomically necessary. A breath taken in a collapsed position engages the upper chest, not the diaphragm. A breath taken in an open position, with the shoulder blades retracted and the rib cage expanded, engages the diaphragm from its designed position and produces the full vagal stimulation that makes the breath neurologically meaningful. Many breath practices fail to produce their intended effect because they ask for the breath without first creating the postural conditions for it.
>
> **Breathe** third, with the long exhale, to initiate the vagal stimulation that begins shifting autonomic balance. The extended exhale is the key element—six to eight counts out compared to four counts in—because it is the exhale, not the inhale, that stimulates the vagus nerve. This is the parasympathetic trigger. One breath, in the open-chested position that precedes it, through a cervical spine that has been repositioned, produces a

neurological event that would not have been possible in either the collapsed position or without the preceding structural adjustment.

Expand fourth, lifting the gaze above the horizontal, because the visual mode shift changes the cognitive and attentional state in ways that the postural and respiratory changes alone do not produce. The panoramic gaze activates the default mode network, softens the sympathetic activation associated with narrow focus, and creates the neurological conditions for the broader, more creative, more socially available mode of consciousness that the contracted state suppresses. The Expand element transforms the Twenty-Second Lift from a physical practice into a complete state change—addressing body, breath, and attention simultaneously.

Move fifth, briefly, to consolidate the change through the motor system and break the postural holding pattern that the contracted state produces. A shoulder roll, five steps, a gentle spinal rotation—any of these signals to the nervous system through a different channel: movement. The body that moves is telling the nervous system something different from the body that is still. Movement creates safety. Movement is capacity. Movement is the signal that the threat the contracted posture was responding to has resolved and the system can return to its designed state.

A final note on sequence. After the Move element, some practitioners add a closing moment of PAIN—one more beat of awareness, noticing what has changed in the body during the twenty seconds. The opening PAIN reads the body before the practice. The closing PAIN reads what the practice accomplished. A growing number of practitioners add one more element to this closing beat: a small, genuine smile. The instruction is simple—as you complete the Lift, let a soft smile form. This is not decoration. Experimental work by Tara Kraft and Sarah Pressman, published in *Psychological Science* in 2012, found that people who held a smile during a stressful task recovered faster physiologically, with lower heart rates during recovery, than those who held a neutral expression[3]—an effect strongest for the genuine, eye-engaging Duchenne smile.

The facial-feedback pathway runs both directions: Just as feeling safe produces a smile, forming a smile sends the nervous system a signal of safety. Ending the Lift with a smile tells your own physiology that you are safe, present, and connected—the precise autonomic message the whole practice is built to deliver. Over weeks and months, the closing PAIN is what develops the reader's sensitivity to their own physiological signals—the capacity to feel, with precision, the difference between the regulated state and the unregulated one. That sensitivity is how a reader stops needing to understand the practice intellectually. They know it from the inside.

Seven elements. Twenty seconds. The sequence compounds because each element creates the conditions for the next. Perform them out of order and the effect is reduced. Perform them in sequence and the effect is the whole that is greater than the sum of its parts.

Making It Permanent: The Trigger-Behavior Pair

Behaviors attached to existing triggers persist far more reliably than behaviors that must be independently remembered. This is not a motivational observation—it is a neurological one. The brain is a prediction machine. When a trigger reliably predicts a behavior, the behavior becomes automatic. The goal is automaticity, not discipline.

Choose your triggers. Every time you pick up your phone. Every time you open your laptop. Every time a meeting ends. Every time you sit down or stand up. The pairing need not be exhaustive—two or three consistent trigger-behavior pairs, practiced without exception, will accumulate to dozens of daily lifts by the end of the first week.

By the end of the first month, the body begins to anticipate the trigger. The lift starts before the phone is in the hand. That is the moment the practice has become an identity. That is the moment you have become someone who looks up. There is an even simpler way to hold the whole practice in mind. The aspiration is a Twenty-Second Lift roughly every twenty minutes you are awake—which works out to about one minute, three times an hour, spent regulating the one system that runs everything else. Said another way: one minute per hour, invested in yourself. Framed as a percentage, it is less than 2 percent of your waking time given to the nervous system that determines the quality of the other 98 percent. When the practice is described as a thirty-day program or a new discipline, it can feel like one more thing to fail at. When it is described as one minute per hour—sixty seconds to tune in and tune up the most important system you own[4]—it becomes what it actually is: the most attainable health habit available to any human being with a spine and a breath.

Sophia Stops Needing to Understand It

Sophia Jones is forty-seven and has been a middle school principal for nine years, which means she has spent nine years managing other people's emergencies from seven in the morning until five in the evening, then driving home to manage her own family's needs from five thirty until ten. She describes herself as a person who does not have room for one more practice in her life, which may be entirely accurate. She does not have room to add a practice to her life. She does have room for twenty seconds.

The distinction matters. When Sophia's clinician suggested the Twenty-Second Lift, her first response was the response of every person who has tried and abandoned meditation apps, journaling rituals, morning routines, and evening reflection practices: "I'll try it, but I'll probably forget." She had not forgotten the other practices. She had run out of the margin they required. A practice that asks for a dedicated window of time is asking a person like Sophia to create something she does not have, time. A practice that attaches to something she is already doing is asking for nothing extra. Just a different quality of attention at an existing moment.

Sophia carries a two-way radio. Most principals do. It is the tool that reaches her for every crisis, every visitor at the front door, every student who needs to be called to the office. She picks it up twenty to thirty times per day without thinking about it. That is twenty to thirty existing triggers, already firing reliably, already anchored in her daily pattern.

Her clinician suggested one pairing: Every time she picks up the radio, she does the Lift first. Not after. Before. Three seconds of spinal extension, one open breath, gaze lifted and widened. Then she answers.

"Twenty seconds seems insultingly small," she said. "It feels like it shouldn't count."

Two weeks later, Sophia says: "I still don't fully understand why twenty seconds works. But I'm done needing to understand it. It works."

What works, specifically: The three o'clock wall that had been her most reliable companion for nine years had noticeably diminished. Her husband mentioned, unprompted, that she seemed less wired when she got home. Her sleep—always fragmented in the way that school administrators' sleep tends to be, interrupted by early-morning anxiety about the day ahead—had improved. She attributed all of this to the radio trigger.

What she was observing was the compound effect of twenty to thirty brief autonomic resets distributed across a day. Each reset is too small to notice individually. The aggregate is measurable across weeks. This is how the minimum effective dose functions at scale: not through any single application but through the accumulation of applications so small and so frequent that they change the baseline from which the nervous system operates without the person ever experiencing the change as an effort.

By month two, Sophia told her clinician something that surprised them both: "I notice now when I miss it. If I grab the radio too fast, without the Lift, it feels different. The conversation goes differently. I'm less patient. I respond more than I think."

This is the marker that matters most. Not the self-reported improvement in sleep or the husband's observation or the diminished afternoon wall. The moment

Sophia could feel the difference between the regulated state and the unregulated one—the moment she had enough contrast to notice the absence of what the practice provided—is the moment the practice had become an identity. She was no longer someone trying to do the Lift. She was someone who does it, who knows what it gives her, and who notices when it is missing.

That is not a program. That is life.

Key Takeaways:

- The Twenty-Second Lift is the minimum effective dose for state change—the smallest intervention that produces reliable, immediate neurological effect.
- Autonomic shifts begin within seconds of postural change because the proprioceptive pathways are rapid and the brain stem's response is immediate.
- The seven elements—the practice of PAIN, Lift, Open, Breathe, Expand, Move, and a closing practice of PAIN with a gentle smile—are sequenced to compound each other's neurological impact.
- Habit formation requires pairing the Lift with existing triggers, not relying on independent memory or motivation—the goal is automaticity, not discipline.
- By the end of the first month, the body begins to anticipate the trigger—that is the moment the practice has become an identity.

Put It into Practice

Choose three triggers from today—three things you will already do, without exception. Attach the Twenty-Second Lift to each of them. Not as a rule. As a pairing: When this happens, I do that. Write them down. Do them today, without exception. Do them again tomorrow. On day three, notice whether your body has begun to anticipate the trigger before it arrives. That anticipation is your nervous system learning a new normal.

CHAPTER 7

The Look Up Day

Morning, Evening, Technology, and Movement

A single lift is a moment. A day built around looking up is a different life.

Individual practices are powerful. A day designed around them is transformative.

This chapter gives you the full architecture of a Look Up Day—from the first moment of waking through the last moment before sleep. Not a rigid schedule that demands perfection, but a framework of principles that flexes to the reality of your actual life while still delivering the consistent physiological inputs your nervous system requires.

Morning: Breathe Before You Screen

The most important rule of the Look Up Day is this: Do not touch your phone until you have done three things. Lift your head. Open your chest. Take ten full breaths.

That is the morning alignment. It sets the neurological baseline from which your entire day unfolds. Every notification, every email, every decision you face will be processed by a nervous system that starts from expansion rather than contraction if you give it those ninety seconds first.

Maya tried this for the first time on a Tuesday. She left her phone face down on the nightstand, sat at the edge of the bed, and took ten slow breaths before she reached for it. Then she stood and moved her spine—reaching overhead, rotating left and right, folding forward, and returning—for two minutes.

Then she looked out the window at the sky, which was gray and unremarkable. For thirty seconds she just looked at it. Let her eyes travel as far as the distance would allow. Took three more full breaths from that expanded gaze.

Then she reached for her phone.

The First Three Minutes

The most consequential minutes of the Look Up Day are not the ones you spend exercising. They are not the ones you spend meditating, or journaling, or reviewing your intentions for the day. They are the first three minutes after you open your eyes.

Here is why. The autonomic nervous system does not enter waking from a neutral state. It enters waking from sleep, which for most people means it has been in a period of reduced sympathetic activity and has the potential to set its waking baseline from a relatively clear starting point. What happens in the first three minutes of waking—the first sensory inputs, the first postural positions, the first breath patterns—begins calibrating that baseline. It is a moment of unusual plasticity, and most people spend it in the worst possible way: reaching for a phone.

The research on morning cortisol response is relevant here. The cortisol awakening response—the spike in cortisol that occurs in the first thirty minutes after waking—is a normal and necessary hormonal preparation for the day. Its amplitude is influenced by what the person does upon waking. Exposure to social threat stimuli (which is what most social media content consists of, at a neurological level) elevates the cortisol awakening response. Exposure to natural light, movement, and slow breath lowers it. The first choice of the day—phone or not-phone—is a hormonal choice, a neurological choice, a choice about what kind of physiological foundation the rest of the day will be built on.

Maya's first morning practice was not dramatic. She sat at the edge of her bed—not the floor, not a meditation cushion, just the edge of the bed—and took ten slow breaths. Ten breaths, approximately ninety seconds. She kept her eyes closed for the first five and open for the last five, letting the morning light in her bedroom register gradually rather than all at once.

On the first morning, she almost stopped after three breaths. The pull of the phone was specific and physical—not a vague distraction but a clear bodily orientation toward the device on the nightstand. She had not realized, until that moment, how strong that orientation was. How trained it was. How much of her first conscious experience every morning had been organized around the small rectangle of glass and light that had become, without her choosing it, the first thing her nervous system encountered every day.

She told her clinician later that the most surprising part was not how different she felt—though she did feel different, clearer in some way she could not yet name—but how much she had resisted those few minutes. How loud the pull toward the phone had been. "It made me realize," she said, "how much of my morning I had been giving to something that was not giving me anything back."

Three minutes is what it costs to begin every day from a different neurological starting point. The day that builds from that starting point is not a different day in any external way. The schedule is identical. The demands are identical. The work is identical. But the nervous system processing all of it begins from expansion rather than contraction. And expansion, sustained across the day by the trigger-paired Lifts and the movement snacks and the evening alignment, compounds. Not dramatically. Not overnight. The way interest compounds: quietly, consistently, and eventually in ways that cannot be predicted from any single deposit.

Maya had felt, for the first time in years, like the day belonged to her—even if only for those three minutes before it didn't.

Technology: The Three Principles of Conscious Use

- **Bring technology to you:** Stop bending your body toward your devices and start positioning devices to meet your body. Monitor at eye level—the top third of the screen at or slightly below the horizontal eyeline. Phone held at or above the horizontal when possible. This single structural change reduces forward head posture mechanically, continuously, without requiring any ongoing attention or willpower.
- **Interrupt the accumulation:** No posture, however optimal, should be sustained for ninety minutes without interruption. Set an interruption threshold—we recommend forty-five to sixty minutes—and at that threshold, stop, stand, perform the Twenty-Second Lift, and move before continuing. The interruption need not be long. Twenty seconds is the floor, not the ceiling.
- **Balance narrow focus with expansion:** For every sustained period of close-range screen engagement, create a brief period of its opposite—far gaze, wide visual field, open awareness. The 20/20/20 principle—every twenty minutes, look at something twenty feet away for twenty seconds—is the practical form of this principle, serving both eye health and nervous system regulation simultaneously.

Movement: The Snack Schedule

Movement snacks are brief, frequent inputs of movement variety distributed throughout the day—the practical solution to the body's need for positional variation within the reality of a workday that demands sustained desk presence. Four patterns are most suppressed by sedentary screen work and most urgently needed:

- **Spinal extension:** reaching overhead, opening the chest, gently arching the upper back—the direct countermovement to the collapse

- **Spinal rotation:** gentle left and right turns, holding each end range for a breath—restoring the rotational capacity that sitting progressively removes
- **Hip extension:** standing exercises that stretch the front of the hip (for example, a standing lunge with the back leg straight, or stepping one foot back and pressing the hips gently forward)—addressing the hip flexor shortening that prolonged sitting produces and that alters walking mechanics, lower back health, and upright posture over time
- **Lateral movement:** side-bending reaches in each direction—activating lateral stabilizers that are entirely absent from sedentary work patterns

The minimum effective schedule: one-minute movement snacks every forty-five to ninety minutes, a five-minute walk every three hours, and one ten-minute full-movement practice somewhere in the day. That is, at most, thirty minutes of distributed movement across an eight-hour workday. The return—in cognitive performance, physical comfort, and afternoon energy—far exceeds in value the time it requires.

Evening: The Threshold Before Sleep

The thirty minutes before sleep are as consequential as the ninety seconds after waking, and for the same reason: The nervous system at the boundaries of the day is in a state of relative openness to recalibration. The morning threshold sets the baseline from which the day proceeds. The evening threshold sets the conditions from which sleep proceeds—and sleep, as Matthew Walker's research has comprehensively documented,[1] is when the nervous system performs the maintenance that determines the quality of the next day's function. What you do in the thirty minutes before sleep shapes the quality of that maintenance.

The specific problem with screen use before bed is not primarily the blue light spectrum—though that is a real and documented factor in circadian disruption. The more significant problem is the neurological state that screen engagement produces and maintains. The sympathetically activated, narrowly focused, informationally dense state of engaged screen use is essentially the opposite of the state the nervous system requires to make the transition to restorative sleep. You cannot shift from that state to sleep efficiently. The system needs a physiological bridge—a transition period in which the inputs change from activating to settling.

Maya discovered this by accident. She had been following the morning alignment for three weeks when she noticed, on a Wednesday, that she had fallen asleep faster than she could remember having done in years. She had not done anything differently that evening. Except that she had left her phone on the kitchen counter when she went to bed, because she was too tired to carry it, and had instead lain on the floor for two minutes doing the evening breath sequence from this chapter—not deliberately, but because she had read it that morning and it was on her mind.

The two minutes on the floor. The ten slow breaths. The one acknowledgment—she named the moment that afternoon when her daughter had shown her a drawing and she had genuinely looked at it and said something true about what she saw. Then she lay in bed and was asleep, she estimated afterward, within six minutes.

She has since made the floor practice nonnegotiable. Not every element. Not the full extended version. Two minutes. Ten breaths. One thing that was real today. The specificity matters: not a gratitude list, not a reflection journal, not a review of the day's accomplishments. One moment. Named. The nervous system receives that as a signal: The day had value. The vigilance required to protect that value is no longer needed. Recovery can begin.

The research on presleep practices and sleep quality is consistent in finding that brief physiological settling practices—slow breathing, mild body relaxation, intentional transition from activating activity—improve sleep onset and the proportion of deep sleep achieved. The Look Up evening alignment is a specific application of this research, designed around the postural and respiratory pattern most disrupted by the Heads-Down World and most restorative to correct before sleep. It costs two minutes and a section of floor. The return compounds every morning you wake up more restored than you would have been.

The last thirty minutes before sleep are as physiologically consequential as the first thirty minutes after waking. The nervous system's transition from waking activity to restorative sleep is not automatic—it requires the right conditions. Modern screen use in the hour before bed provides almost none of them.

- **Screen away at least fifteen minutes before your target sleep time**. Not primarily because of blue light—because the postural and neurological state of screen engagement is incompatible with the parasympathetic dominance that restorative sleep requires.
- **Floor position.** Two minutes, lying on your back, knees bent, feet flat. Ten slow breaths—longer exhale than inhale. Let the floor take the weight you have been carrying all day. This is not stretching. It is the physical equivalent of setting something heavy down.
- **One acknowledgment.** Before sleep: Name one moment from today when you were present, capable, or connected. Not a gratitude list. One thing. A regulatory signal to the nervous system: The day had value. Recovery can begin.

The Breath Tool Kit

The breath tool kit in this chapter is not a collection of breathing exercises. It is a set of neurological tools, each calibrated for a specific physiological objective. Understanding the mechanism behind each one is what makes the tool kit reliable under pressure—because the person who knows why a tool works reaches for it at the right moment, rather than the person who has memorized a technique but does not know what problem it solves.

The physiological sigh deserves special attention because it is the fastest single-breath intervention documented in the current research literature. Andrew Huberman and colleagues at Stanford identified the physiological sigh as the fastest way to offload carbon dioxide from the bloodstream—and it is excess CO2, more than low oxygen, that is a primary driver of the physiological anxiety response.[2] The two-part inhale through the nose—a first inhale to fill the lungs, a brief pause, a second short inhale to reinflate any collapsed alveoli—followed by a long slow exhale through the mouth is not a mindfulness practice. It is a respiratory intervention with a documented mechanism, a measurable effect, and a timeline measured in seconds. One breath. The fastest physiological reset available.

The six-breaths-per-minute resonance frequency is the second most important tool in the kit, and the most important for the transition to sleep. The cardiovascular system has a natural resonant frequency—the rate at which the heart's own oscillation and the breath's rhythm are in maximal synchronization. For most people, this is approximately six breaths per minute: five counts in, five counts out.

At this rate, heart rate variability is maximized, vagal tone is at its highest, and the autonomic nervous system is as parasympathetically dominant as it can be in the waking state. Research by Richard Gevirtz and colleagues at Alliant International University has documented that even brief practice at resonance frequency produces measurable improvements in HRV and subjective relaxation.[3] Ten minutes before sleep brings the nervous system to the most favorable possible starting point for the transition to restorative rest.

The activation breath—the rapid full-cycle breathing followed by the exhale-hold—is the most counterintuitive tool in the kit because it involves deliberate hyperventilation, which most people associate with anxiety rather than performance. The key is what follows: The exhale-hold produces a brief CO2 buildup that, paradoxically, produces calm rather than anxiety in most individuals, followed by a deep inhale and hold that floods the system with oxygen and produces what many practitioners of this activity describe as a clear, energized, alert state without any sympathetic activation.

This is the activation breath's specific value: clarity and energy without the agitation that caffeine or sympathetic stimulation produces. Use it for low-energy mornings, midday slumps, or any moment when you need to access your best cognitive function without the anxiety that typically accompanies urgency.

- **Activation (low energy, low focus):** Twenty-five rapid, full inhales and exhales through the nose, then a breath-hold on empty, then a deep inhale held for fifteen seconds. Use for morning or midday energy restoration.
- **Regulation (stress, anxiety):** Inhale four counts, exhale eight. Five minutes produces a measurable parasympathetic shift. Use before difficult interactions or after stressful events.
- **Immediate reset (acute stress):** The physiological sigh—two quick inhales through the nose to fully inflate, followed by a long slow exhale through the mouth. The fastest single-breath stress intervention identified in current research.
- **Sleep transition:** Six breaths per minute—five counts in, five counts out. This is the cardiovascular resonant frequency, the rate at which heart rate variability is maximized. Ten minutes before sleep improves sleep onset and deep sleep proportion.

Key Takeaways:

- Breathe before you screen: Ninety seconds of deliberate physiological alignment before engaging with devices sets the neurological baseline for the entire day.
- The three principles of conscious technology use—bring technology to you, interrupt the accumulation, balance narrow focus with expansion—address the interface problem without requiring abstinence from technology.
- Movement snacks—brief, frequent, targeting the four patterns most suppressed by sedentary work—provide distributed sensory nutrition throughout the day.
- The evening alignment—screen away, floor position, one acknowledgment—sets the conditions for restorative sleep and determines the physiological starting point of the next morning.
- Four breath protocols serve four distinct physiological objectives: activation, regulation, immediate reset, and sleep transition. Having the right tool for the right moment is more effective than a single approach applied uniformly.

Put It into Practice

Design tomorrow using this framework. Write down your morning alignment (ninety seconds before the phone), three trigger-paired Twenty-Second Lifts, your movement snack schedule, and your evening alignment. Not a wish list—a specific plan, attached to specific triggers and times. Then do it. The day after, do it again. By day seven it will no longer feel like a plan. It will feel like your day.

CHAPTER 8

Look Up at Work

The Workplace as a Physiological Environment

You do not just work in your environment.
Your nervous system is shaped by it, hour after hour.

The average knowledge worker spends forty to fifty hours per week in their workplace. In that time, the physical environment they occupy—the chair, the desk height, the monitor position, the lighting, the acoustic conditions, the cultural expectations around movement and stillness—shapes their physiological state as powerfully as anything they deliberately practice.

You can do the Twenty-Second Lift ten times a day and still spend the hours between those twenty-second interventions in an environment systematically generating Tech Posture Syndrome. Which is why this chapter is not optional.

The Culture of Stillness Is Costing You

The equation of stillness with productivity is not an ancient cultural value. It is a relatively recent artifact of the industrial and then knowledge-work economy, and it was never designed with the biology of the knowledge worker in mind. It was designed around the economics of factory production, in which physical stillness genuinely did correlate with output: A worker who was still was usually operating a machine, and a worker who was moving was not. The equation was applied to office work without examination, and it persists in knowledge work without examination, even though knowledge work has a fundamentally different relationship with the body than machine operation does.

The research on attentional recovery—developed by Kaplan and Kaplan's Attention Restoration Theory in the 1980s and replicated across dozens of subsequent studies[1]—established that directed attention, the kind required for sustained cognitive work, is a resource that depletes with use and requires specific conditions for recovery.

Those conditions include what Kaplan calls "fascination"—engagement with something that captures interest without demanding directed attention, which natural environments consistently provide, and screen environments consistently do not. The knowledge worker who walks to a window and looks out for thirty seconds is not taking a break from cognitive work. They are performing the restoration that makes the next twenty minutes of cognitive work possible.

The organizations that have figured this out—and the research on high-performing teams consistently identifies them—are not the ones with the most rigorous productivity policies. They are the ones with the most sophisticated understanding of how human attention works, and the cultural permission for their people to manage their attention as a resource rather than a virtue. The leader who takes a visible movement break is not modeling a lax attitude toward work. They are modeling the physiological intelligence that distinguishes sustained high performers from the people who burn bright for two years and then quietly begin declining.

Modern professional culture has, without ever examining the assumption, equated stillness with productivity. The person who stays seated and screen-focused for eight uninterrupted hours is understood to be working hard. The person who stands periodically, walks to a window, or takes a movement break is understood to be not working.

This assumption is not merely wrong. It is demonstrably, measurably counterproductive. The brain is not a machine that performs better with more continuous operation. It is an organ with specific recovery requirements—attentional cycles of approximately twenty to fifty minutes followed by brief recovery periods—and the failure to meet those requirements produces cognitive performance declines that accumulate across the afternoon and compound across years.

The high performers in knowledge work are not the ones who move the least. They are the ones who have learned—sometimes intuitively, sometimes deliberately—to manage their physiological state across the workday rather than simply grinding through it.

Why Ergonomics Failed—And What Works Instead

The ergonomics movement addressed the right problem with the wrong solution. It recognized that office environments were causing musculoskeletal injury and sought to correct the interface between human bodies and work equipment. Adjustable chairs, wrist rests, monitor stands, lumbar supports: The intervention portfolio grew impressively.

And yet musculoskeletal disorder rates in screen-based occupations have not fallen as ergonomic adoption has risen. The reason: Classical ergonomics tried to find the optimal static position and sustain it. But the human body does not thrive in any single position, however optimal. It thrives in movement—in the continuous, low-level, varied physical activity that the Heads-Down World has systematically removed.

The highest-leverage ergonomic change for most desk workers is not a better chair. It is a monitor raised to eye level. This single change—which costs nothing beyond the inconvenience of stacking books or adjusting a stand—reduces forward head posture mechanically and continuously, without requiring any ongoing attention. It is the change with the largest postural return for the smallest investment. Do it before you finish this chapter.

The Look Up Workday Model

State-Based Scheduling—The Performance Multiplier

Of all the Look Up Workday interventions, state-based scheduling produces the largest cognitive return per unit of attention invested, because it changes not just the content of what the knowledge worker does but the physiological conditions under which they do it.

The research on cognitive performance across the day is remarkably consistent across different study populations and methodologies. Complex, creative, high-stakes cognitive work—the work that requires the prefrontal cortex to be operating at its full capacity, with adequate blood flow, well-rested attentional resources, and high HRV—is best performed in the two to three hours following peak alertness. For most chronotypes, this window falls in the mid-to-late morning. It is also, for most knowledge workers, the window most frequently consumed by email, administrative tasks, and the meetings that are scheduled at nine because nine was available.

The executive who schedules emails or routine informational meetings at nine a.m. because the calendar is open is making a catastrophic physiological mistake dressed as an administrative decision. They are using their highest-quality cognitive resource—the window of peak prefrontal function that will not recur until the following morning—on the lowest-stakes, most easily automated, most interruptible tasks in their day. And they are using the afternoon, when prefrontal function has declined and administrative inertia is the only fuel still available, to attempt the creative strategy work or the complex analysis that deserves their best.

State-based scheduling inverts this. Complex, creative, highest-stakes work goes in the morning window. Administrative, reactive, interruptible work goes in the afternoon. Meetings—which consume attention without primarily requiring the kind of deep prefrontal focus that generates original thinking—go in the transition periods. The knowledge worker who structures their day this way is not working harder. They are working in alignment with the physiological reality of how their brain functions across the day.

The Look Up Practice amplifies this alignment. The morning alignment that begins the day from a regulated physiological baseline extends the effective window for high-quality cognitive work. The movement snacks that interrupt accumulated postural load prevent the cognitive decline that sets in at the ninety-minute mark without recovery inputs. The Twenty-Second Lifts distributed across the day maintain the HRV and prefrontal blood flow that support sustained cognitive performance. The evening alignment that creates the conditions for restorative sleep ensures that the next morning's window begins from the highest possible baseline.

The compound effect of state-based scheduling plus the Look Up Practice is not additive. It is multiplicative. The person who is in a better physiological state and who is doing their best work during their best physiological window is not performing 20 percent better than the person who is in an average physiological state doing their best work at the wrong time. They are performing in a category that is not directly comparable to the depleted, mistimed alternative. The quality of output that emerges from peak physiological state at peak cognitive time is qualitatively different—more original, more integrated, more surprising to the person producing it—than the competent output that emerges from an adequate physiological state at an adequate time.

This is the multiplier that no productivity system addresses. Every productivity system optimizes within the system as it is. State-based scheduling, combined with the physiological practices that create the state worth scheduling around, optimizes the system itself.

- **Alignment anchors:** The Twenty-Second Lift performed at specific transition points—beginning and end of day, before and after meetings, at the midpoint of any sustained focus block. Nonnegotiable. Twenty seconds each.
- **Movement intervals:** Positional change every forty-five to ninety minutes. Standing, a movement snack, a brief walk. This interrupts the accumulation that generates postural and cognitive deficits.
- **Visual breaks:** Three to five moments per day of deliberate far-gaze—thirty to sixty seconds of looking into the distance, eyes soft, peripheral field active. These restore visual mode balance and provide brief but meaningful nervous system regulation.

- **State-based task scheduling:** Complex, creative, or high-stakes work scheduled for peak state windows—typically midmorning for most people. Administrative and reactive tasks scheduled for natural lower-energy periods. The quality of knowledge work is determined not only by time on task but by the physiological state of the person doing it. This is the performance multiplier that no productivity system addresses.

For Leaders: The Most Powerful Lever Is Free

The most powerful single organizational intervention is not structural—it is cultural. And cultural change follows one path: leadership modeling.

If senior leaders take movement breaks visibly and without apology, movement breaks become normalized. If leaders begin meetings with sixty seconds of physiological alignment—"let's take one minute before we start"—that practice spreads. If executives raise their monitors to eye level and their teams can see it, monitor adjustment rates in the organization rise.

You cannot mandate your way to a physiologically healthy workplace. You can model your way there. And the modeling costs nothing except the willingness to be seen doing something that matters.

The ROI case is documented: Research consistently finds that unhealthy employee behaviors—sedentary lifestyle chief among them—are associated with productivity losses of approximately two thousand dollars per employee per year. In a knowledge-based organization of any size, the return on physiological investment is substantial. But the leaders who understand this do not need the ROI case. They have felt the difference themselves. That is where every cultural change in this area begins.

The Workplace of the Future—Five Years from Now

Imagine what the leading knowledge-work organization looks like in five years, if it takes the physiological argument of this book seriously.

The headquarters has a certified Human Doctor on-site two days per week—not an occupational health physician treating injuries after they occur, but a vitality practitioner whose entire mandate is nervous system optimization before dysfunction appears. Employees book fifteen-minute sessions during the workday for spinal assessment, HRV baseline review, and the kind of hands-on care that no app or algorithm replicates.

The practitioner knows each employee's physiological patterns the way a performance coach knows an athlete's training data. The sessions are not a perk. They are a performance investment in the same category as the standing desks, the ergonomic chairs, and the meditation room, except this one has sixty years of peer-reviewed clinical science behind it and produces measurable changes in the upstream variable that determines what all the other interventions can accomplish.

The Human Doctor has made a recommendation—logged in the employee's vitality record, not their medical file—that they transition their primary mobile computing interface to a heads-up device for tasks that do not require sustained fine-screen work. The recommendation is clinical, not corporate: Based on the employee's postural assessment and HRV baseline, sustained forward head posture is the primary driver of their afternoon cognitive wall and their chronically low sleep quality scores. Reducing the mechanical load on their cervical spine during mobile computing hours will address both. Here is the device. Here is how to use it. Here is what we will measure at your next session to confirm it is working.

This is what it looks like when the Human Doctor model meets the heads-up computing revolution in a workplace context. The medical doctor prescribes pharmaceutical tools to achieve physiological targets. The Human Doctor prescribes technological and behavioral tools to achieve vitality targets. Both are clinical recommendations. Both are grounded in assessment, measurement, and follow-up. Only one of them addresses the cause rather than the symptom. Only one of them makes the employee more capable rather than merely more managed.

The organization's HRV dashboard—aggregated and anonymized, measuring workforce nervous system regulatory capacity as an organizational metric alongside revenue and Net Promoter Score (NPS)*—shows a trend that has been moving upward for eighteen months. Absenteeism is down. Cognitive performance scores, measured through validated task completion rates in the company's project management system, are up.

The afternoon productivity wall that used to flatten output between two and four p.m. has largely disappeared. The leadership team attributes it, in their annual report, to the investment in workforce physiological health. The CFO attributes it, more precisely, to the fact that eliminating the cognitive cost of Tech Posture Syndrome in a workforce of three thousand people recovered approximately six million dollars per year in previously invisible productivity losses—at a program cost of less than $300,000.

This is not speculation. Every component of this vision exists today. The Human Doctor Institute is training the practitioners. The heads-up computing devices are available at consumer scale. The HRV measurement technology is in the wearables already on employees' wrists. The productivity data already exists

* Net Promoter Score is a market research metric that is based on a single survey question asking respondents to rate the likelihood that they would recommend a company, product, or a service to a friend or colleague.

in every organization's project management system. The only missing piece is the framework that connects these components into a coherent model of organizational vitality—and a leader willing to build it. That leader is reading this book right now.

Key Takeaways:

- The workplace is the primary environment in which Tech Posture Syndrome is created and sustained—making it the highest-leverage point for intervention.
- Professional culture's equation of stillness with productivity is empirically false and actively counterproductive to the cognitive performance it claims to support.
- Classical ergonomics failed by treating a dynamic problem as a static one—the answer is not the optimal position but the maximum variety of positions.
- Raising the monitor to eye level is the single highest-return ergonomic intervention for most desk workers—do it before you finish this chapter.
- Leadership modeling is the highest-leverage organizational intervention—culture follows what senior people are seen doing, not what policy documents require.

Put It into Practice

Today, raise your monitor to eye level. If you do not have a monitor stand, use books. Measure: When seated in your normal working posture, the top third of your screen should be at/or slightly below the horizontal eyeline. Work from this height for the rest of the day and notice how much less effort it requires keeping your head up. Then, at your next meeting—whether you are leading it or attending—say: "Before we start, let's take sixty seconds." Open your posture, take three slow breaths, look away from screens. Note the quality of what follows.

CHAPTER 9

Looking Up in Relationships

The Most Personal Cost

The people we love most are the ones who notice first when we are looking down.

There is a moment that Maya knows well.

It happens at the dinner table, usually around six thirty. Mia is telling her something—about school, about her friend Jasmine, about something she saw on the way home—and Maya is listening. She is nodding. She is asking the right questions in the right places. She is, by every observable measure, present.

And yet.

There is a quality of attention that Maya knows she is capable of—a depth of presence she can feel herself giving at her best—and she can feel, in the subtle gap between what she is offering and what she knows is possible, that she is not fully engaged. That Mia is getting the performance of her mother's attention rather than her full undivided attention.

Mia has not said anything. As a reminder, she is only nine. She does not have the vocabulary for what she is sensing. But she is sensing it. Children always do.

What Full Presence Actually Requires

The research on attunement—the quality of synchronization between two people's physiological and emotional states that characterizes genuine relational presence—has consistently found that it is not a psychological achievement. It is a biological one. The nervous systems of two people in genuine attunement show measurable convergence in their physiological signatures: HRV patterns, cortisol rhythms, vocal prosody, and the timing of micro-expressions that signal the tracking of another person's internal state. This convergence is not something either person is doing deliberately. It is something their nervous systems are doing automatically, given the right physiological conditions.

Those conditions require the ventral vagal state in both parties. A person in sympathetic activation—however well-intentioned, however skilled at conversation, however committed to being present—cannot achieve the depth of attunement that the ventral vagal state makes possible. They can have a conversation. They can be in the room. They can say the right things. The convergence—the quality that makes another person feel genuinely seen and met rather than merely heard and responded to—is not fully available.

This has specific implications for every significant relationship in a life that includes sustained knowledge work. The person who arrives at a dinner table after ten hours of sympathetically activated screen engagement is physiologically limited in their capacity for the quality of presence that dinner tables with people they love are supposed to provide. Not permanently. Not irreversibly. But in that moment, before any physiological preparation has been made, the depth of attunement available is constrained by the state of the nervous system doing the attuning.

The threshold practice changes this by doing one specific thing: It creates a brief window in which the autonomic state can shift before the new context begins. Twenty seconds is not enough to fully recalibrate from a dysregulated day. But it is enough to begin the shift—and beginning the shift, rather than walking directly from one context into another with no physiological transition, produces a measurable difference in the quality of presence available on the other side of the threshold.

The difference Maya's daughter feels at the dinner table is not in the content of what her mother says or does. It is in the quality of the nervous system meeting her—whether the social engagement circuits are fully operational, whether the facial expressivity and vocal warmth and genuine tracking of what she is saying are available at full capacity. Children feel this difference before they can name it. Partners feel it before they can describe it. The quality of presence is its own communication, independent of any word spoken, and it arrives through channels that no amount of trying harder can access. It arrives through the physiological state of the person entering the room.

Genuine human presence—the kind that makes another person feel truly seen—is not a psychological achievement. It is a physiological one. It requires a body that is open, a nervous system that is regulated, a visual system that is fully engaged with the human face in front of it rather than still calibrated for an eighteen-inch screen, and a breath that is not constricted.

A person who has spent ten hours in Tech Posture Syndrome is not neurologically or physiologically capable of their best relational presence when they walk through the door. Their postural system is still oriented toward the screen. Their nervous system is still in its slightly contracted, slightly vigilant mode. Their social engagement circuits—the ventral vagal system dedicated to reading faces, interpreting vocal tone, and synchronizing physiological state with another person—are available but depleted.

This is not a character flaw. It is a physiological state. And physiological states are changeable.

Elena's Two Minutes

Elena Reyes was forty-three, a hospital administrator and mother of three children aged eight, eleven, and fourteen. She was, by any fair accounting, doing everything right: present at the school play, at the soccer games, at the dinner table every night she possibly could be. And she knew, with a clarity that troubled her, that present was not the same as being here.

"I'm always managing something from my last location," she told us. "Even when I'm home, part of me is still at work. My kids feel it. I feel it. I just don't know how to make the transition actually happen."

She began one practice: Before pulling into her driveway each evening, she sat in the car for two minutes. Phone face down. Eyes closed. Five full breaths—long, slow exhales. One spinal rotation each direction. Then she walked in the door.

The first night, her eight-year-old daughter said: "Mom, you seem different tonight."

She had not changed anything else. Same day. Same stress. Same traffic. Two minutes in the car.

"That's when I understood," Elena told us. "I'd been trying to be present through willpower. I didn't understand that presence is a physiological state. You cannot simply will your way into it. You have to create the conditions for it."

The Threshold Practice

> *You cannot give what your nervous system does not have. The practices in this book are not just for you. They are for everyone who needs the best version of you to show up.*

The relational application of the Look Up Practice is the threshold practice: Before engaging with a person who matters to you—before the meal, the conversation, the reunion at the end of a workday—give your nervous system twenty seconds to complete its transition.

Sit in the car. Pause at the top of the stairs. Stand outside the door for one breath. Do the Twenty-Second Lift. Let the screen-calibrated visual mode soften. Let the contracted state begin to release. Then cross the threshold.

This is not about arriving perfect. It is about arriving deliberately, intentionally. The goal is not to be untouched by the day you've had—it is to choose, actively, to enter the next context from a different physiological state than the one you are carrying.

Maya tried this on a Wednesday. She sat in the parking garage of her building for ninety seconds before going upstairs. Paid attention inside. Lifted, opened, breathed, expanded, moved. Took one more breath, noticed what had changed, and let a small smile form. Then she went to her door.

Mia met her in the hallway. And for the first time in longer than Maya could precisely remember, she felt herself arrive.

The Neuroscience of Presence

What Elena experienced in the car—and what her eight-year-old daughter immediately noticed—is not mysterious when viewed through the lens of polyvagal theory. It is the predictable consequence of a brief but deliberate shift in autonomic state, applied at the moment of transition between two physiological contexts.

Stephen Porges's research identified what he called the social engagement system: a set of neurological structures, primarily mediated through the ventral vagal complex, that enable the specific quality of face-to-face engagement that human beings require for genuine connection.[1] This system controls facial expressivity, vocal prosody, the ability to read micro-expressions, and the physiological synchronization between two people in genuine attunement—the phenomenon sometimes described as being on the same wavelength, which turns out to have a literal autonomic correlation.

Critically, the social engagement system is fully operational only in the ventral vagal state. It is suppressed in sympathetic activation. A person who has spent ten hours in the physiological state that Tech Posture Syndrome produces—elevated sympathetic baseline, reduced vagal tone, compressed respiratory function—is arriving at their family with a social engagement system that is available but not fully operational. They are physiologically capable of interaction. They are not physiologically in the state from which their deepest interactions proceed.

This is what Elena's daughter felt. Not the absence of love, but the absence of the specific physiological signature that signals to another nervous system: I am here, fully, and I am safe to be with. Children's nervous systems are exquisitely tuned to this signal. They read it in the quality of the parent's voice, the openness of their facial expression, the fluidity of their movement, the depth of eye contact. They read it before any word is spoken. And they respond to its presence or absence in ways that shape their experience of being loved.

The two minutes Elena spent in the car were not a meditation. They were a physiological preparation—the deliberate creation of the autonomic conditions under which her social engagement system could operate at full capacity. Her daughter felt the difference before Elena had finished closing the door.

Key Takeaways:

- Full relational presence is a physiological achievement, not merely a psychological one—it requires a regulated nervous system, open posture, and a visual system recalibrated from screen to person.
- The social engagement circuits of the autonomic nervous system operate from the expansion state—genuine attunement at the depth that makes people feel truly met requires physiological conditions, not only intention.
- Children are exquisitely sensitive to the quality of parental physiological presence—they feel the gap between performance and the real thing before they have words for it.
- The threshold practice—twenty seconds of deliberate physiological transition before engaging with the people you love—is one of the highest-return investments described in this book.
- Presence is a physiological state, not a character quality. You cannot simply will your way into it. You create the conditions for it.

Put It into Practice

Tonight, practice the threshold. Before you engage with anyone you love after a period of work—whether walking through a door, sitting down at a table, or picking up a phone for a personal call—take twenty seconds first. Lift, open, breathe, expand, move. Then cross the threshold. Observe what happens in the first five minutes of that interaction compared to what usually happens. Then observe whether they notice. You may be surprised how quickly another person's nervous system recognizes when yours has shifted.

What has the other person in the relationship noticed?

This follow-up signals to the patient that the relational domain is as clinically important as the structural one—which it is—and that you are tracking their progress in the process with the same rigor you track their postural improvement.

PART III
THE FUTURE

A New Model of Care—and the Technology That's Finally Catching Up

CHAPTER 10

Why Healthcare Is Failing

The Missing Piece

Modern medicine is brilliant at naming what has already broken.
It rarely asks why the system stopped regulating itself.

Maya has seen her doctor six times in the past two years. Blood work, thyroid panel, sleep study, referral to a therapist, referral to a physical therapist for the neck. Each visit generated a bill. Each bill addressed a symptom. None of them addressed the cause.

This is not a criticism of her doctor, who is competent and caring. It is a description of a system designed—at its foundations, in its economics, in its training, in its measurement—to respond to illness rather than to maintain health. A system that is extraordinarily good at catching people after they fall and largely unprepared to help them not fall in the first place.

The Downstream Trap

Modern medicine excels at acute intervention. Surgical techniques once unimaginable are now routine. The pharmacological management of acute illness has saved lives on a scale that staggers the imagination.

And yet, by the measures that matter most to most people—the experience of daily health, the quality of functional life across decades—the system is failing. Ninety percent of healthcare spending in the United States goes toward managing chronic conditions with primary causes that are behavioral and environmental. The system is spending its $4.5 trillion overwhelmingly downstream: treating the consequences of problems that, at an earlier stage, could have been addressed for a fraction of the cost.

Tech Posture Syndrome illustrates this gap with acute precision. It is not a disease, so it generates no diagnosis code. Its symptoms—fatigue, anxiety, brain fog, chronic musculoskeletal pain—are real and significant, but they are managed individually while the structural pattern generating all of them goes unaddressed. Maya leaves each appointment with a new intervention for a symptom. She has never once been assessed for the upstream cause.

The Nervous System Revolution

There is a quiet revolution underway in the scientific understanding of health—one accumulating evidence at a pace that will eventually make its influence unavoidable.

The revolution concerns the nervous system. Specifically: the recognition that the nervous system is not merely the communication infrastructure of the body but its primary coordinator of health, function, and adaptation across every other organ system. And that the state of the nervous system is not merely a consequence of health or illness—it is a determinant of it.

Dr. Stephen Porges's polyvagal framework, developed across three decades of research, has been particularly clarifying: The state of the autonomic nervous system actively determines the body's capacity for immune function, cardiovascular regulation, digestive efficiency, hormonal balance, and tissue repair.[1] A nervous system chronically operating in threat states does not simply feel bad. It is physiologically compromised in ways that generate, sustain, and worsen physical illness.

This means that addressing nervous system state—directly, as a clinical objective in its own right—is a legitimate and powerful healthcare intervention, one that most current healthcare practice is structurally unprepared to offer.

The Spine as Neural Infrastructure

Dr. LaMarche's story is the most personal illustration of why this matters clinically. The subluxations in his upper spine—C7 to T4—were not causing musculoskeletal pain. They were disrupting the neurological signals to his heart and lungs. The correction of those subluxations restored the signals. The system responded. His heart returned to normal size.

The principle is the same for Maya, for Daniel, for every person experiencing the diffuse and confusing symptom cluster of Tech Posture Syndrome. The postural distortion in the upper cervical and thoracic spine is not primarily a structural problem. It is a neurological one. It is disrupting the proprioceptive signals that calibrate the autonomic nervous system—and the consequences of that disruption manifest throughout the body in ways that standard diagnostics are not designed to detect.

What gets measured gets managed. The health system measures disease. It does not yet measure nervous system regulatory capacity—the upstream variable that determines health and the physiological experience of daily life.

The Direction Modern Medicine Is Running

It is worth being specific about what "the future of medicine" looks like from the inside of the institutions building it—because the direction is not ambiguous, and understanding it is essential for understanding why the Human Doctor model is not a supplement to that future but an essential.

Major health systems across the United States and Europe are actively deploying remote patient monitoring programs that track biometrics—blood pressure, glucose, heart rate, oxygen saturation, medication adherence—continuously and algorithmically. The stated goal is earlier intervention: Catch the deviation from the normal range before it becomes a crisis. This is, within its own logic, a reasonable objective. But the logic itself deserves examination.

The model being built is one in which the patient is primarily a data source. Their body generates readings. Algorithms compare those readings to population-derived baselines. Deviations trigger alerts. Alerts trigger protocols. Protocols specify interventions—most commonly pharmacological. The physician in this system is increasingly a gatekeeper between the patient and the algorithm, executing protocols rather than practicing clinical judgment. The patient's role is to be compliant: to take the medications, to maintain the metrics within the specified range, to generate readings that do not trigger alerts.

This model is extraordinarily sophisticated at one thing: detecting pathology. A blood glucose reading that drifts above a threshold will be caught faster, and responded to more consistently, than in any previous era of medicine. That is genuinely valuable. For acute conditions, for infectious disease, for the management of established chronic illness—the algorithmic model has real and documented benefits.

But the model has a structural blind spot so large it encompasses most of what makes a human life worth living. It has no instrument for vitality. It has no measurement for the experience of being fully alive—energetic, focused, resilient, present, growing. A person whose metrics are all within normal range may be experiencing exactly what Maya was experiencing: persistent fatigue, fractured focus, shallow sleep, the persistent low-grade wrongness of a nervous system that has been held in an incorrect position for years. Every algorithmic check in that person's medical record says "No intervention required." The patient experiences something different. The model has no category for the gap.

Monitoring your biometrics to determine when your blood chemistry requires pharmaceutical intervention is not going to create vitality. It is going to create compliance. And compliance—with a normal range defined by population averages and managed by algorithmic alerts—is not the same thing as health. It is the management of the absence of measurable disease. These are categorically different objectives. Only one of them produces a life worth living.

> The future of medicine is AI monitoring your compliance with the absence of disease. The future of health is you paying attention to the presence of your own vitality. These are not the same future—and only one of them requires a human being.

We want to be precise about what we are and are not arguing. We are not anti-medicine. Medicine saves lives every day in emergency rooms, operating theaters, and intensive care units around the world. The acute care model—the one medicine was designed for—is among the most consequential achievements in human history. A person having a stroke needs a neurologist, not a chiropractor. A person with bacterial sepsis needs antibiotics administered by a physician who knows exactly what they are doing.

The argument is more specific: Medicine's acute-care model—built on pharmacological intervention triggered by deviation from a baseline—has been exported into the chronic disease and preventive health space, where it does not belong and does not work. Chronic pain managed with opioids. Anxiety managed with benzodiazepines. The diffuse malaise of Tech Posture Syndrome managed with . . . nothing, because no diagnosis code exists for it. And now the algorithmic monitoring infrastructure being built will automate and accelerate this pattern—not out of malice, but because the model it is automating was never designed to generate vitality. It was designed to detect and suppress pathology. Faster. At scale. With less human contact at every step.

Again, we are not anti-medicine. We are pro-vitality. And those are not the same position.

The Financial Case for Getting This Right

The argument for the Look Up approach is not only physiological. It is economic—and the numbers are large enough that they belong in any serious conversation about the future of healthcare and organizational performance.

The United States spends approximately $4.5 trillion ($4,500,000,000,000.00) per year on healthcare. Ninety percent of that spending goes toward managing chronic conditions with primarily behavioral and environmental causes. Musculoskeletal conditions—the category that most directly captures the downstream consequences of Tech Posture Syndrome—are among the leading drivers of disability and lost productivity in the developed world.

The United States Bone and Joint Initiative has estimated that musculoskeletal conditions cost the United States approximately $213 billion per year in treatment, care, and lost wages (based on 2011 data).[2] The Global Burden of Disease study consistently ranks neck pain and low back pain among the top causes of years lived with disability worldwide. These are not small numbers. They are the financial fingerprint of a civilization that has been looking down for fifteen years.

The cognitive cost is harder to quantify and almost certainly larger. A knowledge worker operating at 80 percent of their physiological capacity—due to chronic nervous system dysregulation, respiratory restriction, and the postural compression that Tech Posture Syndrome produces—is delivering 80 percent of the output their organization is paying for. Every day. Invisibly. With no diagnosis code, no sick day, no insurance claim.

The Health Enhancement Research Organization has documented that employees with high health risks cost organizations approximately two thousand dollars more per year in health care costs than their healthier counterparts—and that figure does not capture the cognitive dimension, which research consistently shows to be the most economically significant consequence of physiological underperformance in knowledge work.[3]

Now consider the cost of the alternative. The Twenty-Second Lift takes twenty seconds and costs nothing. A movement snack program for an organization of one hundred people requires no equipment, no external vendor, and perhaps thirty seconds of a senior leader's time at the start of each meeting to normalize it. A monitor raised to eye level costs a stack of books. The upstream intervention—the one that addresses the cause rather than managing the consequence—is free. The downstream intervention—the pharmacological management of symptoms that were generated by a postural and neurological problem that was never addressed—costs $213 billion a year and rising.

The financial case for getting this right—for investing in the upstream, for organizing healthcare around the support of vitality rather than the management of pathology—is not a close call. It is perhaps the largest unrealized return available to any organization, health system, or government that is willing to ask the question the current system is not designed to ask: not what is wrong with our people, but what would they be capable of if we gave their nervous systems what they need?

The most expensive thing in the modern economy is a human being operating at a fraction of their capacity. The least expensive intervention is twenty seconds. The choice between these futures is not a close call—financially, physiologically, or humanly.

There is a deeper problem still. The healthcare system has trained people to interpret their body's signals as threats to be eliminated rather than communications to be read. A headache is not a Tylenol deficiency. Fatigue is not a caffeine deficiency. Anxiety is not a benzodiazepine deficiency. These are the body speaking—in the only language available to it—about inputs it requires and is not receiving.

The body speaks in whispers before it screams. Tech Posture Syndrome begins as a whisper—a slight tightness, a fatigue that lingers, a focus that frays. When those whispers are suppressed rather than read, they escalate. The whisper becomes chronic pain. The chronic pain becomes functional limitation. The functional limitation becomes the defining experience of a life. And the medical system, organized around treating the scream, never addresses the conditions that generated the whisper in the first place.

The alternative is what we call proactive PAIN: Pay attention inside now. Not as a crisis response—but as a practice. A daily, deliberate orientation toward the signals the body is sending, before they escalate. A healthcare system built on PAIN would not wait for the scream. It would cultivate the capacity to hear the whisper—and to respond with the inputs that make the escalation unnecessary.

There is a name for the paradigm this chapter has been describing. It is the painkiller paradigm—the cultural and economic orientation that treats symptoms as problems to be eliminated rather than as information to be acted upon. The painkiller paradigm generates a predictable cascade: Signals are suppressed, the underlying conditions continue to deteriorate, the suppressed signals escalate, and eventually the body produces a crisis that can no longer be silenced. At that point the system intervenes with surgery, injection, or higher-dose pharmaceutical management. Every step of this cascade is expensive. Every step imposes its own physiological costs. And none of it addresses the original whisper that could have been responded to, years earlier, at a fraction of the cost and without any of the side effects.

The pain detector paradigm—the orientation this book has been teaching—is the alternative. It is the discipline of receiving signals at the whisper stage, responding to them with the inputs the body is asking for, and making the escalation unnecessary. A healthcare system organized around the pain detector paradigm would look different from the one we have. It would cost less. It would produce more. The people inside it would be healthier. The shift from the first paradigm to the second is not a medical revolution. It is a philosophical one—and the practices in this book are how an individual makes the shift inside their own life, regardless of what the surrounding system does.

That is the system this book is trying to build. One person, one practice, one whisper heard in time.

Two of the most prominent voices in the current public conversation about technology and health are worth placing in direct relationship to this argument. Jonathan Haidt's research in *The Anxious Generation* establishes, with epidemiological rigor, the scale of the adolescent mental health crisis that followed smartphone adoption.[4] He tells us how many people are affected and how severely. Tristan Harris, through the Center for Humane Technology, has documented the design intent behind the engagement-maximizing features that drive the crisis—the infinite scroll, the notification architecture, the algorithmic amplification of activating content. He tells us why the platforms were built the way they were built.[5]

What neither of them fully addresses is the mechanism—the specific physiological pathway through which the harm operates in the body. Tech Posture Syndrome is that mechanism. The forward head, the collapsed chest, the compressed diaphragm, the reduced vagal tone, the elevated sympathetic baseline: This is the physical architecture that the Heads-Down World builds inside every person who inhabits it, and it is the architecture that makes everything Haidt and Harris document more severe. A dysregulated nervous system does not just scroll more—it scrolls differently, engaging with threat content more readily, generating the engagement signals that teach the algorithm to serve more threat, in a feedback loop that operates at the body level before it reaches the level of conscious choice.

When the Algorithm Is Wrong

The clinical case for why the algorithmic monitoring model fails for Tech Posture Syndrome is worth making precisely, because it illustrates a structural problem that will become more consequential as AI-mediated healthcare expands.

The algorithmic model begins with a diagnostic category. If the patient's presentation matches the criteria for the category, the algorithm assigns the diagnosis and specifies the treatment. If it does not match, the algorithm finds no diagnosis and specifies no treatment, or specifies "watch and wait," or specifies symptom management.

Maya's presentation does not match any diagnostic category. Her fatigue does not meet the criteria for chronic fatigue syndrome. Her anxiety does not meet the criteria for generalized anxiety disorder. Her neck pain, when she reports it, is managed with ibuprofen and does not generate a referral to any practitioner who might assess its structural origin. Her cognitive difficulty does not meet the criteria for any attentional disorder. She is, in diagnostic terms, a person with subclinical findings across four domains, none of which individually triggers the algorithm's response threshold.

The upstream problem—the forward head posture, the compressed diaphragm, the reduced HRV, the postural pattern that is generating all four subclinical findings simultaneously through a single mechanism—is not a diagnostic category. There is no ICD-10 code for Tech Posture Syndrome. There is no reimbursement pathway for assessing it. There is no algorithm that combines neck tightness, afternoon fatigue, ambient anxiety, and brain fog into a single upstream cause, because no diagnostic framework exists to make that combination legible as a pattern rather than four separate subclinical complaints.

The AI system being built by healthcare organizations to improve care efficiency will, if it is built on the current diagnostic framework, make this problem worse. It will identify patterns—that is what AI does well—but it will identify patterns within the diagnostic categories that exist. Maya's four subclinical complaints will generate four AI-identified management recommendations, none of which addresses the upstream cause, and none of which would individually be wrong. The AI will not be failing. The framework will be.

The Human Doctor model bypasses this problem by asking different questions. Not "which diagnostic category does this presentation match?" but "what is the state of this person's nervous system, and what structural and environmental factors are driving that state?" These questions generate an assessment that no current AI can perform, because it requires integrating information from a lateral posture photograph, a breath pattern observation, an HRV measurement, a patient history of daily technology use and movement patterns, and a hands-on spinal assessment—and synthesizing those into a clinical picture that the reductionist diagnostic framework was never designed to represent.

This is the Human Doctor's irreplaceable contribution: the ability to see the whole person and the upstream variable that coordinates the whole person's experience, in a way that no algorithm built on the current diagnostic framework can replicate. Not because AI is incapable of integration—AI is extraordinary at integration within its training domain—but because the training domain of current healthcare AI is disease categories, not vitality states. And disease categories are the wrong map for the territory Maya is actually in.

That is what the Human Doctor model exists to address.

The Invisible Patient

The medical system's failure to address Tech Posture Syndrome is not a failure of individual practitioners. None of them failed her in the way we normally mean when we say a clinician failed a patient. They all did what they were trained to do.

The failure is structural. It is built into the design of the system that trained them.

Modern medical training organizes knowledge around diagnosis codes. A patient presents with a cluster of symptoms. The clinician maps those symptoms to a diagnostic category. The diagnostic category specifies a treatment protocol. The treatment protocol is executed. This sequence works well for a patient who has something the diagnostic categories were designed to detect: an infection, a fracture, a named chronic disease, a measurable deficiency.

It fails systematically for a patient whose primary presenting experience is a diffuse reduction in functional capacity that has no diagnostic code. Fatigue that is not anemia. Brain fog that is not hypothyroidism. Anxiety that is not panic disorder. Musculoskeletal pain that is not a discrete injury. The experience is real, significant, and measurably impairing—and the diagnostic system has no container for it. So the clinician does what the system trains them to do: Rules out the named diagnoses, documents that the workup is unremarkable, and writes "manage your stress."

This is not malpractice. It is the logical output of a system designed to find specific named things, applied to a patient who has something the system was not designed to find. The problem is the design.

The Human Doctor model is, at its foundation, a different design. Not a replacement for diagnosis—diagnosis remains essential when something specific and named is present. But a complement to it: a clinical framework organized around the question the current system never asks. Not "which named category does this patient's experience fall into?" but "what is the state of the upstream system that coordinates this patient's entire physiological experience, and what does that system need to function at its best?"

The upstream system is the nervous system. The answer to what it needs is documented in the research this book cites. And the practice of providing it—through spinal adjustment, postural correction, breath rehabilitation, movement restoration, and the education that allows the patient to maintain what the clinician initiates—is what the Human Doctor does.

Maya does not need a better diagnosis. She needs the answer to a different question. This book is that answer, delivered in the form she can use.

Key Takeaways:

- Modern medicine excels at acute intervention but was designed to respond to illness rather than maintain health—90 percent of healthcare spending goes toward managing chronic conditions whose causes are behavioral and environmental.
- Tech Posture Syndrome illustrates the system's structural failure. It is a clinically significant syndrome with no diagnosis code, whose individual symptoms are treated while the root cause goes unaddressed.
- The polyvagal revolution establishes that nervous system state actively determines immune function, cardiovascular regulation, hormonal balance, and tissue repair—making nervous system care a legitimate primary clinical objective.
- The spine is neural infrastructure: The functional state of its joints and tissues directly influences the proprioceptive signals that calibrate the autonomic nervous system.
- The health system measures disease. It does not yet measure nervous system regulatory capacity—the upstream variable that determines the physiological quality of daily life. The Human Doctor model exists to fill this gap.

Put It into Practice

Before your next healthcare appointment—routine or otherwise—prepare three questions no clinician has ever asked you in a clinical setting:

- How is my posture affecting my nervous system function?
- How is my breathing pattern affecting my stress resilience and anxiety?
- What in my daily physical environment is contributing to my symptoms?

Bring the questions with you and ask them. The quality of the response will tell you immediately whether you are receiving care organized around function or around symptoms—and whether you are in the right clinical relationship.

CHAPTER 11

The Human Doctor

A New Model of Care

The future of care is not a better disease manager.
It is a partner in keeping you well.

The Human Doctor is not a credential. It is a philosophy—and a standard of care that differs from the disease-management paradigm in several fundamental ways.

A Human Doctor does not wait for pathology to appear. They work at the level of function: assessing how well the system is working before asking what is wrong with it and intervening to optimize that function rather than merely suppress symptoms.

A Human Doctor centers their care and interventions around the nervous system. They understand that the regulatory capacity of the nervous system is the primary upstream variable for most of the health outcomes their patients care about, and they address that capacity directly.

And a Human Doctor educates. They do not simply treat—they transform the patient's relationship to their own body. A patient who leaves a Human Doctor's care knowing why their posture matters, how their breath regulates their nervous system, and what their daily movement patterns are doing to their long-term health has received something that will outlast the specific intervention. They have received understanding. And understanding compounds.

The Power of Hands-On Care

There is something that no algorithm replicates, and that the science of human healing is increasingly clear about: the therapeutic effect of skilled human physical contact.

What Cannot Be Automated

The discussion of AI in healthcare often proceeds as though the only question is speed and accuracy: Can the algorithm diagnose faster and more accurately than the clinician? This question, while important, misses the most significant dimension of what clinical care should provide.

A skilled clinician's hands provide information that no sensor currently replicates. The quality of tissue under manual assessment—its tone, its temperature differential, its movement quality, its response to gentle loading—conveys information about the state of the nervous system that drives those tissues. A palpating clinician who has developed their tactile sensitivity through years of practice can identify the pattern of neurological facilitation in the paraspinal muscles before any imaging finding supports it, can feel the qualitative difference between protective muscle guarding and primary dysfunction, can distinguish by touch the joint that is hypermobile from the one that is fixated in a way that no current objective measurement captures at the clinical scale.

Beyond the information the clinician's hands receive is the information they transmit. Therapeutic touch—skilled, intentional, calibrated contact applied to a nervous system in need of recalibration—activates the C-tactile afferent system, a slow-conducting network of skin nerve fibers tuned specifically to gentle, human-speed touch,[1] the oxytocin pathway, the autonomic nervous system's response to safe physical contact in ways that no algorithmic intervention can replicate. The patient who lies on an adjustment table in a well-trained clinician's office is receiving a physiological experience that no telemedicine platform, AI coaching interface, or wearable sensor can provide.

This is not a romantic defense of traditional practice against technological progress. It is a precise claim about the mechanism. The neurological effects of skilled human touch operate through pathways that require physical contact. Those pathways were built over millions of years of evolution in social species whose nervous systems learned to regulate in the presence of other bodies. They are not a legacy system waiting to be replaced. They are the primary system—the system that technology should be building around, not attempting to replace.

The Human Doctor understands this. They embrace technology as a tool for extending their clinical intelligence—the biometric data that illuminates patterns invisible to observation, the imaging that confirms what palpation suspects, the AI coaching that supports the patient between visits. But they do not confuse the tool for the practice. The practice is the relationship between a skilled human nervous system and a patient's nervous system, mediated through clinical training, genuine attention, and the irreplaceable information exchange of physical contact.

That relationship cannot be automated. It can be augmented. It can be made more effective with better data. It can be extended to more people more efficiently. But at its center, it requires a human being who has developed the clinical capacity to perceive what the patient's nervous system is doing and to respond with the specific, calibrated input that moves it in the right direction. That is what the Human Doctor does. It is what no algorithm currently does, and it is what no algorithm in the foreseeable future is likely to do.

Heal the Ouch with Touch

There is a phrase that captures what this chapter has been describing in clinical language, and it comes not from a research paper but from the accumulated wisdom of a profession that has been saying it in a thousand different ways for 130 years: Heal the "ouch" with touch.

The ouch is real. The neck that aches after ten hours of screen time. The low back that protests the commute. The headache that arrives reliably at two in the afternoon. The diffuse wrongness that has no name and no diagnosis and no pharmaceutical target. These are not imaginary. They are not exaggerated. They are the body's communication—whispers that have been building toward screams—and they are asking for something specific. Not a pill that suppresses the signal. Not an injection that numbs the area. Touch. Skilled, calibrated, human touch, applied by a practitioner who has spent years developing the clinical sensitivity to perceive what the nervous system is doing and to respond with the input that moves it in the right direction.

> Chiropractors are putting the health and the care back into healthcare. Not through a new drug, a new device, or a new diagnostic algorithm. Through the oldest clinical tool available to a human being: the skilled, attentive, fully present encounter between one nervous system and another. That is what the Human Doctor offers. That is what no algorithm currently does, and what no algorithm in the foreseeable future is likely to do.

The Tune-In and Tune-Up

The language people use to describe a practice shapes how we relate to it. When they say we are "going to the chiropractor," the implicit frame is reactive: Something is wrong and it needs to be addressed. When we say we are going for our Tune-In and Tune-Up, the frame shifts completely. Not reactive. Proactive. Not waiting for the ouch. Paying attention before the ouch arrives.

The tune-in is the first half of every skilled clinical encounter, and it is the part that the medical model almost never has time for. Before the adjustment, before the assessment, before any clinical intervention—the question: How are you, really? Not the surface answer. The actual answer. What has the week been like in your body? Where are you carrying it? What has your nervous system been signaling that you have been too busy to fully hear? The tune-in is PAIN practiced with clinical support: Pay attention inside now, with a skilled practitioner as your guide.

The tune-up is what the practitioner's hands do with what the tune-in reveals. The spinal adjustment that addresses the structural finding. The soft tissue work that releases the compensatory holding pattern. The breath cue that restores the diaphragmatic function the posture has been compromising. The specific, calibrated clinical input that moves the nervous system from where it is to where it is capable of being. Together, the tune-in and the tune-up are not a treatment visit. They are a ritual of proactive physiological maintenance—the regular, consistent investment in the upstream variable that determines the quality of every downstream experience.

The person who has a Tune-In and Tune-Up weekly, or every two to four weeks, is not waiting for their body to break down and then seeking repair. They are maintaining the instrument through which they experience their entire life. They are investing upstream, consistently, in the nervous system that coordinates their cognition, their emotion, their resilience, their capacity for presence, and their physiological aging trajectory. They are practicing, in the most literal sense, what this book has been arguing from its first page: that the gap between where most people are and where they are capable of being is not a medical problem. It is a maintenance problem. And maintenance, unlike repair, is inexpensive, pleasant, and available before anything goes wrong.

Find your Human Doctor. Book the appointment. Show up not with a complaint but with the question: What does my nervous system need right now that it has not been receiving? Let the tune-in answer it. Let the tune-up address it. Do this consistently, for months and then for years, and watch what the compound interest of that investment produces in your physiology, your relationships, your work, and the quality of the decades ahead.

Touch is not merely pleasant. It is biologically necessary—a form of sensory input the nervous system processes through dedicated neural pathways distinct from those processing verbal or visual information. Appropriate therapeutic touch activates oxytocin release, reduces cortisol, lowers heart rate and blood pressure, and modulates autonomic nervous system activity in ways that support the shift from sympathetic to parasympathetic dominance.

No algorithm produces these effects. No screen mediates them. They require a skilled human hand, responsive in real time to the tissue it is working with, guided by training and experience and the irreducibly human capacity for attunement.

The evidence base for spinal adjustment in musculoskeletal conditions is substantial, with effect sizes comparable to pharmaceutical management and a substantially superior safety profile. But the evidence most relevant to this book concerns the neurological effects: Research using neuroimaging and autonomic measurement has documented that spinal adjustment produces immediate changes in brain activity and measurable changes in autonomic balance. The spine is not merely being moved. The nervous system is being influenced.

Personal PAIN and Clinical PAIN

The Twenty-Second Lift is PAIN in its personal form. You perform it yourself, many times a day, in the spaces where formal care is not available. You pay attention to your own signals. You deliver your own response. Over months, you become the instrument of your own physiological regulation.

The Tune-In and Tune-Up is PAIN in its clinical form. You perform it with a skilled Human Doctor, periodically, in the space where deeper diagnostic and therapeutic capacity is available. The practitioner pays attention to signals you cannot fully read from the inside. Their hands deliver a response your own hands cannot give yourself. Over months and years, they become a partner in your regulation—an outside perspective on a nervous system that cannot always perceive itself accurately.

These are not two separate practices. They are two forms of the same practice. The personal PAIN is the daily discipline. The clinical PAIN is the deeper maintenance. The personal PAIN builds the self-literacy that makes the clinical encounter more precise and more valuable. The clinical PAIN provides the structural adjustments and calibrated inputs that the personal practice cannot generate on its own. Each makes the other more effective. Neither is complete without the other.

A person who runs the personal PAIN check-in daily and establishes a ritual to Tune-In and get Tuned-Up with a hands-on Human Doctor every two to four weeks is doing what this book has been arguing for from its first page. They are maintaining the instrument through which their entire life is lived. They are investing upstream, consistently, in the nervous system that coordinates their cognition, their emotion, their resilience, their capacity for presence, and their physiological aging trajectory. They are, in the most literal sense, paying attention inside now—and paying for the expert attention that deepens what their own attention cannot reach.

This is the full practice. Personal PAIN (pay attention inside now) every day. Clinical PAIN on a schedule. The Twenty-Second Lift practiced on your own, moving your head, neck, and shoulders. The Tune-In and Tune-Up from the hands of someone trained to do what your hands cannot. Together, they are how a human being stays fully alive in a world that is actively compromising the nervous system through which that aliveness is experienced.

What Peak Performers Already Know

The research confirms what some of the world's highest-performing individuals have been practicing for decades. The connection between spinal health, nervous system function, and peak performance is not a new idea in elite sport. It is an established part of how serious athletes manage their most important asset: their body's capacity to perform under pressure and recover fully from demand.

Michael Jordan—six-time NBA champion, regarded as the greatest basketball player of all time—is described as crediting regular chiropractic care with improvements that extended beyond the physical. "I didn't know how much I could improve until I started seeing a chiropractor," he is widely quoted as saying. "Since I've been in chiropractic, I've improved by leaps and bounds both mentally and physically." That pairing—mental and physical—is not incidental. It reflects exactly what the neuroscience of spinal adjustment is beginning to document: that the benefits extend into cognitive clarity and nervous system regulation, not only into structural function.

Tom Brady—who played elite professional football into his mid-forties, defying every conventional expectation about athletic decline—made chiropractic care a nonnegotiable component of his wellness routine throughout his career. "As long as I see the chiropractor, I feel like I'm one step ahead of the game," he has reflected. The longevity that made Brady the most decorated quarterback in NFL history did not come from any single intervention. But the proactive, systemic approach to physical maintenance that chiropractic represents—not waiting for pain but tending to function before function deteriorates—was central to how he managed his body across two decades at the highest level.

Usain Bolt—the fastest human ever measured and a six-time Olympic gold medalist—dealt with scoliosis throughout his career and turned to chiropractic care as a primary recovery and performance tool. The combination of structural correction and nervous system support that chiropractic provided is described as central to how he managed his condition while competing at the highest level.

Arnold Schwarzenegger, across a career spanning elite bodybuilding, Hollywood action films, and the governor's office of California, has put it simply:

"What chiropractors do is really powerful. I found out the best way is to use chiropractors, not only after injury, but also before injury."

These are not endorsements collected for marketing purposes. (A note on these quotations: While widely circulated and consistently attributed to these athletes across many years, they appear in secondary collections rather than in a traceable primary interview; we present them as popularly attributed rather than as verified on-the-record statements.) They may be observations made by people whose careers depended on understanding, with unusual precision, what kept their bodies performing at the highest level over the longest possible period.

The pattern across them is consistent: Chiropractic care is most valuable not as a pain remedy but as a maintenance practice—a regular input that keeps the nervous system organized, the spine mobile, and the body operating closer to its designed capacity. That is exactly what the Human Doctor model is built on. And it is, in the most direct sense, the application of proactive PAIN—paying attention inside now, before the whisper becomes a scream.

The Adjustment—Why This Word Belongs to Everyone

There is a word that has been quietly controlled by the chiropractic profession for 130 years. That word is "adjustment." We want to give it back.

Inside chiropractic, an adjustment means a specific technical procedure—a high-velocity, low-amplitude manipulation of a spinal joint, performed by a trained clinician. That technical definition is precise, and it is a legitimate part of what this book is arguing for. But the word "adjustment" is much larger than the procedure, and the larger meaning is the one this chapter wants to make visible.

The body is adjusting constantly. Every breath is an adjustment—the diaphragm responds to oxygen demand and changes its rate and depth accordingly. Every heartbeat is an adjustment—the autonomic nervous system reads blood pressure, metabolic need, and emotional state, and calibrates cardiac output in real time. Every step you take is an adjustment—proprioceptors in your feet and ankles send signals to your brain stem, which adjusts muscle tension, balance, and gait from one footfall to the next. The body is not static. It is a continuous process of adjustment, performed by the autonomic nervous system and mediated through hundreds of interlocking biological systems, which is the literal definition of being alive.

The mind is adjusting constantly. Every thought is an adjustment of attention. Every shift in mood is an adjustment of emotional state. Every choice made in response to circumstance is an adjustment of direction. The mind, like the body, is not static. It is a continuous process of adjustment.

The awareness is adjusting constantly—and this is where the reader has agency. The body and the mind adjust automatically. The awareness adjusts by choice.

The decision to pay attention inside now is an adjustment. The decision to move from painkiller mindset to pain detector mindset is an adjustment. The decision to respond to a whisper rather than suppress it is an adjustment. Every time you practice PAIN, you are making an adjustment—a specific, chosen, repeatable adjustment of awareness, which changes the signals your body and mind are operating from.

This is the insight that makes everything the rest of the chapter is saying coherent. When a skilled Human Doctor adjusts a spine, they are not imposing something foreign on the body. They are giving the body's existing adjustment process a specific input it cannot give itself. The adjustment is the body's. The doctor is the catalyst. The skilled clinical adjustment is one valuable form of a universal activity that every living system is already performing, every second of every day, without anyone's conscious involvement.

Adjustments are how you stay alive. They are not interventions performed on you. They are the continuous process by which a living system stays alive. The only question is the quality of the adjustments—whether they bias toward vitality or toward depletion. A person who practices PAIN is making better adjustments of awareness. A person who does the Twenty-Second Lift is making better adjustments of physiology. A person who sees a skilled Human Doctor is receiving adjustments of structure that support both. A life of quality adjustments is a life of compounded vitality. A life of ignored signals, suppressed pain, and neglected structure is a life of compounded depletion. The choice is made in the adjustments, day by day, minute by minute, breath by breath.

There is a physiological principle that gives the cumulative adjustment argument its scientific backbone. It is called allostatic load—the concept, developed by the neuroscientist Bruce McEwen and colleagues, that the body carries the cumulative physiological cost of every stressor it has encountered, and that chronic adaptation to sustained stress produces measurable changes in nervous system regulation, immune function, cardiovascular health, and cognitive performance.

The research is extensive and the mechanism is well-documented. What McEwen's framework makes clear is that the body is not a set of independent systems responding to isolated events. It is a single integrated system, adjusting continuously to a lifetime of accumulated physical, chemical, and emotional inputs, with the cumulative quality of those adjustments determining the quality of the life lived inside the body.

The accumulation runs in both directions. Years of ignored whispers, suppressed signals, and sustained postural compromise accumulate as allostatic load—the body's cumulative cost of chronic neglect. Years of practiced PAIN, consistent Twenty-Second Lifts, regular Tune-Ins and Tune-Ups with a skilled Human

Doctor, and deliberate attention to the inputs the nervous system requires accumulate as something else—the opposite of allostatic load, what we might call allostatic reserve. The compound interest of quality adjustments across a lifetime. The body that, at sixty, is still capable of what most bodies at sixty are not, because the adjustments across the preceding four decades biased toward vitality rather than depletion.

> Adjustments are great things. Make them well. Make them often. Make them yourself in the form of PAIN and the Twenty-Second Lift. Receive them from a skilled Human Doctor in the form of the Tune-In and Tune-Up. Understand that every breath, every choice, every moment of paying attention inside now is an adjustment that shapes the direction of the life the body is carrying you through. The quality of your adjustments is the quality of your life. That is not a metaphor. That is the physiological fact this chapter—and this book—is asking you to act on.

The Human Doctor Institute

Translating this philosophy into clinical practice at scale requires a training framework. The Human Doctor Institute, is that framework.

Certified practitioners complete advanced training in five areas: deep nervous system literacy; applied structural and postural assessment; hands-on clinical mastery; patient education and behavioral change; and the integration of biometric technology with human care. They are practicing a different kind of healthcare—organized around a different question. Not "what is wrong?" but "what is this person capable of, and what does it look like when they are fully alive?"

The Health Span Vision

Chiropractic is the largest drugless health profession in the world. There are more than 100,000 licensed practitioners in the United States and Canada alone, seeing tens of millions of patient visits annually, following a clinical tradition spanning more than a century, built on the premises that the body possesses an Innate Intelligence capable of organizing its own health (the Innate Intelligence of the three-intelligences framework this book develops in chapter 14) and that the practitioner's role is to remove the structural barriers that interfere with that intelligence—not to override it with a chemical or a protocol.

These premises—which the chiropractic profession has held since 1895, often at great cost in terms of mainstream credibility—is exactly what the convergence of neuroscience, autonomic research, and mind-body medicine is now arriving at through different methodological routes. The vitalistic framework was not ahead of its time. It was simply using different language for a truth that the mainstream required a century of peer-reviewed evidence to formally articulate.

As AI accelerates the pathology-detection-and-pharmaceutical-response model of medicine, the counterweight the world needs is already in place. It is organized. It is credentialed. It is present in every community of meaningful size in every country where it has been licensed. It is the only major healthcare profession whose foundational clinical model is not organized around disease but around the support of the body's own capacity for health.

The vital health evolution does not need to be invented. It needs to be claimed—with the confidence that comes from understanding that the science has now arrived at the place the vitalistic tradition has been standing all along. The Human Doctor is not a new idea. It is the oldest idea in healthcare, finally equipped with the language and the evidence to be fully heard.

The healthcare conversation has shifted from lifespan to health span. The concept is James Fries's compression of morbidity: Maximize the period of vigorous functional living, minimize the period of decline.[2] Not more years. More vital years.

Dr. LaMarche is the most personal illustration in this book of what health span looks like when it is actively cultivated. A man who should have died at fifty competing as a gold medalist at seventy, not merely surviving the decades medicine predicted he would not have, but living them at a level of physical capacity that most healthy people decades younger do not approach.

The practices in this book are, in their deepest sense, health span investments. The person who maintains postural integrity, nervous system regulation, respiratory efficiency, and movement variety across their forties, fifties, and sixties is doing something measurably different from the person who does not—preserving the functional capacities that determine whether the later decades are experienced as vitality or as managed decline.

> The Human Doctor's most important question is not "what is wrong with you?" It is "what are you capable of?"—and then, across years of relationship, helping that capability grow.

What Seventy Looks Like from the Inside

The health span argument is abstract until it is inhabited by a specific human life. Dr. LaMarche's life is the most available inhabitation of it in this book—but it is not the only one. The clinical literature is full of patients who, given the right inputs at the right time, have outcomes that standard prognosis did not predict.

The research is consistent: The foundations of functional aging are laid in the decades of midlife. James Fries's compression of morbidity research—first published in 1980 and replicated across multiple datasets since—established that the period of disability and functional decline before death is not fixed. It is compressible. The behaviors and clinical interventions that maintain physiological function across the fourth, fifth, and sixth decades of life do not add years to life. They compress the period of dysfunction into a shorter window at the end, so that the years that were always going to exist are experienced as vitality rather than as managed decline.

This is the Human Doctor's most important gift to their patients: not treating their current condition but changing the trajectory of their physiological aging. A patient who maintains spinal mobility, nervous system regulatory capacity, respiratory efficiency, and movement variety across their forties, fifties, and sixties is doing something measurably different from a patient who does not. The difference does not show up in their annual physical. It shows up in their seventies, when one person is walking their grandchildren to school and the other is managing the consequences of decades of accumulated physiological compromise.

Dr. LaMarche, at seventy-one, is walking evidence of this argument. Not walking evidence that chiropractic care is a panacea—he would be the first to object to that framing. Walking evidence that the nervous system, when properly supported, retains a capacity for adaptation and recovery that standard prognosis does not account for. Walking evidence that the health span conversation is not theoretical. It is personal, specific, and available to every person reading this sentence who is willing to ask not, "What is wrong?" but "What am I capable of?"

The answer to that question, in most cases, is more than the person is currently expressing. The gap between what they are currently expressing and what they are capable of is the space the Human Doctor exists to close.

Key Takeaways:

- The Human Doctor is a philosophy of practice—centering function over pathology, nervous system over symptoms, education over treatment, relationship over transaction.
- Skilled human touch produces specific, irreplaceable neurological effects—activating therapeutic pathways that no digital or algorithmic intervention replicates.
- Spinal adjustment produces documented changes in brain activity and autonomic nervous system function, not merely in musculoskeletal structure.
- The Human Doctor Institute provides the training framework that translates the Human Doctor philosophy into clinical practice at scale.
- The health span model—maximizing functional vitality across the full arc of life—is the ultimate goal of Human Doctor care, and the practices in this book are its daily infrastructure.

Put It into Practice

If you are not currently receiving any form of hands-on care centered on nervous system and spinal health, consider what your system might be experiencing from its absence. Seek a practitioner who discusses nervous system function, not only pain management. Listen for the language of function—vitality, regulation, optimization—rather than the language of pathology alone. That language signals a different model of care, organized around what you are capable of becoming, not only what is currently wrong.

CHAPTER 12

Technology Is Not the Enemy

The Rise of Heads-Up Computing

The device that bent us downward is about to lift our gaze back to the horizon.

This book has spent eleven chapters documenting what technology use, in its current predominant form, does to the human body. It is a serious accounting. But it would be a significant misreading to conclude from it that this book is anti-technology.

The premise is more precise: The problem is the interface between technology and human biology that current device design has produced—an interface that requires the human body to adapt to the machine, rather than the machine adapting to the human.

This is beginning to change. And the change, when it fully arrives, will be among the most consequential developments in human health of our era.

Eleven Billion + Hours Per Day

There are approximately eight billion people on earth. Approximately 3.5 billion own smartphones. Average global smartphone use is now estimated at three to four hours per day—and rising significantly in younger demographics.

That is, conservatively, eleven + billion human hours per day of forward head posture. Of compressed diaphragms. Of narrowed visual fields. Of sympathetic nervous system activation sustained in the absence of any actual threat.

This is not a personal health problem. It is a civilization-wide problem. And its solution cannot come only from individual practice—it requires a structural shift in how the technology interface is designed.

That shift is underway.

The First Interface Designed for Human Biology

For most of the digital era, technology was designed for computation. The keyboard, the mouse, the flat screen: functional solutions to engineering problems, not solutions to the problem of how a human body can interface with computation without paying a physiological price.

Heads-up computing—the emerging category of interfaces that bring computational information into the user's natural forward field of view rather than requiring postural compromise to access it—is the first paradigm in the history of digital technology to treat human biology as a primary design constraint rather than an afterthought.

The forms it takes vary: voice interfaces, smart glasses, heads-up displays, and ultimately full augmented reality. What they share is the essential inversion: The information comes to the human, in the human's natural orientation, rather than requiring the human to bend toward it.

The Companies Building the Way Out

The heads-up computing transition is not a single-company story. It is an industry-wide convergence that is currently underway across the largest technology platforms in the world, with parallel investments in adjacent categories that will determine how the transition unfolds. Naming the participants matters, because the strength of the transition depends on its breadth.

In early 2024, Apple announced and shipped the Apple Vision Pro, a spatial computing device that, while priced for the developer and enterprise market in its first generation, represents the company's strategic commitment to the visual-computing paradigm. Apple's historical pattern is to enter a category at the high end and drive cost and form-factor improvements through subsequent generations. The Vision Pro is the opening move in what Apple intends to be the next major computing platform after the iPhone. The integration of that platform with the Apple Watch, with HealthKit, and with the company's expanding biometric-sensing capabilities means that an Apple-led path through the heads-up future will arrive bundled with the most extensive personal-health-data infrastructure of any technology company.

Meta's investment is the largest single corporate bet on the heads-up computing future, with the Reality Labs division operating at a multibillion-dollar annual investment level for nearly a decade. The Ray-Ban Meta smart glasses described earlier in this chapter are the consumer-scale beachhead of that investment. The Quest line of mixed-reality headsets is the immersive-experience platform. The Orion prototype unveiled in 2024—full augmented reality glasses in a near-consumer form factor—signals where the Meta product line is going. By the late 2020s, Meta intends to ship glasses that deliver smartphone-class computational capability at a form factor comparable to ordinary eyewear. If that ship date holds, the heads-up transition will be a consumer reality within the planning horizon of the average employer reading this book.

Google's historical commitment to the category—going back to Google Glass in 2013 and continuing through the Project Iris and current Android XR initiatives—has been less consistent in product execution but no less consistent in strategic intent. Google's partnership with Samsung on the Android XR platform announced in 2024, and the broader integration of Gemini AI capabilities into wearable form factors, positions Google as the operating system layer for a multi-vendor heads-up future in the same way Android became the operating system layer for the multi-vendor smartphone era.

Snap has shipped multiple generations of Spectacles, currently focused on the developer market, with a sustained commitment to AR as a creative and social medium. Magic Leap, Niantic, and a constellation of smaller players are building enterprise and creative applications that will inform the consumer experience as the platforms mature.

In parallel, the wearable biometric category—currently dominated by Apple Watch, Garmin, Whoop, Oura, Fitbit, and a growing roster of specialist devices—is the sensor-and-data layer that will integrate with the heads-up computing layer to produce what this book has been calling functional support technology. Oura's sustained focus on HRV and sleep architecture, Whoop's on recovery and strain, Garmin's on athletic performance, and Apple Health's on broad longitudinal integration—taken together, these companies have built the measurement infrastructure that the heads-up computing platforms will use to deliver real-time, personalized, physiologically informed coaching at scale.

The hardware exists. The data exists. What is missing is the framework that connects the measurements to the interventions in a way that produces outcomes rather than scores.

That framework is what this book provides. The convergence of these companies, currently uncoordinated, around a shared physiological model of what the human body needs from its computing interface—and what the data those interfaces collect should be used for—is the missing layer that would turn a parallel-investment race into a coordinated industry transformation. We are not naive about the competitive dynamics that make such coordination difficult.

We are not pretending that the companies named above are aligned on anything other than the commercial logic of owning the next computing platform. We are saying that the underlying physiology is the same regardless of which company's hardware delivers the experience, and that the framework in this book is available to any company willing to build the heads-up future around what the human nervous system actually needs.

The companies named above are not adversaries in this story. They are partners—whether they have yet recognized themselves as such or not. The heads-up computing transition will succeed or fail at industry scale, not at single-company scale. Every company building toward the heads-up future is an ally of the human bodies the Heads-Down World has been quietly compromising. The invitation of this chapter is to all of them.

Meta and the Consumer Frontier

The release of the Meta Ray-Ban Smart Glasses in 2023 represented something specific in the history of computing that is easy to understate: It was the first time a major technology company shipped a product whose primary interface is the human voice, directed forward, in normal physical orientation, at consumer scale and at a consumer price point. Previous voice interfaces—Siri, Alexa, Google Assistant—all required the user to direct their attention toward a device to engage them. The Ray-Ban glasses require nothing. You speak. The interface responds. Your head stays where your head is when it is not looking at a screen.

The Oakley HSTN collaboration extended this into the athletic market with the specific design constraints of outdoor sport: polarized lenses, durable frames, open-ear audio calibrated for wind noise, and a form factor that works with helmets, visors, and the physical demands of trail running, cycling, and snow sports. Marcus, who uses both, has observed the difference clearly: The Ray-Bans change his workday, and the Oakleys change his athletic performance. Both change his physiological baseline in ways the book has already described.

What neither product yet does is the next step. Neither has biometric sensing integrated into the temple arms, where PPG measurement is possible. Photoplethysmography (PPG) is a noninvasive optical technique that measures blood volume changes in microvascular tissue using light, typically from LEDs, and a photodetector. It is commonly used in wearables (smartwatches) and medical devices to monitor heart rate, blood oxygen saturation, respiration, and blood pressure by detecting volumetric changes in arteries during cardiac cycles. Neither product has postural detection software that reads the angle of the user's visual field relative to the horizon. Neither delivers real-time HRV-triggered breath guidance through the open-ear speakers. These are the next capabilities—and the companies building this hardware are, by the logic of their own product trajectories, positioned to add them. The hardware exists. The AI coaching architecture exists. The biometric sensing technology exists in other form factors. The integration is a software and sensor problem, not a physics problem.

The company that solves that integration problem will not be selling a wellness product. They will be selling the world's first computing interface that is simultaneously the world's most effective physiological support tool. That is a different value proposition than any wearable device has previously offered. It is also, if this book's argument is correct, the value proposition that the market has been waiting for without knowing it was waiting for it. Because the market has been buying biometric trackers for a decade and the trackers have been providing data without providing outcomes. The next product that provides outcomes—that intervenes at the moment of maximum physiological relevance, with the minimum disruption to workflow, in a form factor the user is wearing anyway—will define the category for the decade that follows.

Meta Ray-Ban Smart Glasses was the first mass-market consumer technology product allowing meaningful computational interaction in a format requiring no postural compromise whatsoever. You wear them. You look forward. You talk to them. They respond. Your head stays up.

This seems like a small thing until you understand what every previous computing interface has required of the human body. Then it seems like an obvious and overdue revolution.

Meta has made augmented reality its primary long-term technological bet—a multi-decade, multi-hundred-billion-dollar commitment to building the interface it believes will eventually succeed the smartphone as the primary computing platform. Apple, Google, and others are pursuing parallel trajectories at comparable scale. Whatever one thinks of these companies, the convergence of investment is significant: The largest technology organizations in the world are collectively betting on a computing paradigm that is, by its inherent structural design, heads-up.

A person interacting with mature augmented reality in an upright, forward-oriented position is not generating forward head posture. Their cervical spine is loaded normally. Their diaphragm has full room to descend. Their visual field is broad. Their gaze is directed forward and slightly upward—precisely the gaze orientation associated in every study we have cited with nervous system expansion, parasympathetic activity, and cognitive breadth.

Technology used in this orientation does not produce Tech Posture Syndrome. It is, in the most literal sense, the difference between looking up and looking down.

A Vision of the Heads-Up Future

Imagine, for a moment, what daily life looks like when the primary computing interface is not in your hand but in your field of vision—ambient, unobtrusive, and structurally aligned with the orientation of a human body at its best.

You wake up and move through your morning alignment with your visual field open and clear—no phone to reach for, no screen to hunch toward. Information comes to you as you stand upright, as you walk, as you look outward at the world. Your notifications arrive at the periphery of your vision and recede without demanding your cervical spine as the price of access. Your calendar, your messages, your navigation—all of it present in the space ahead of you, at eye level, requiring nothing of your posture that your posture was not already giving.

You have a conversation with a colleague, face-to-face, and neither of you looks down once. The information you need floats in your shared visual field—referenced without breaking eye contact, without interrupting the social engagement circuits that both of your nervous systems require to do their best work together. The meeting ends. You walk to your next engagement. You look up. You keep looking up.

Your children grow up in this world. They learn to read on devices that meet their eyes at the right level. They play games that require them to look outward, to move, to engage their peripheral vision and their full bodies. The default posture of their generation is not the question mark that a posture photograph reveals—it is the open, upright, forward-facing orientation of a human being in full engagement with the world around them.

This is not science fiction. It is the direction of technology—and it is a direction that is, for the first time in the history of the digital era, aligned with the direction of the body. That alignment—technology and biology finally moving in the same direction—is among the most consequential developments for human health of the coming decade. And the companies investing in it are not doing so for health reasons. They are doing so because it is where computing is going. The health implications are a gift that arrives alongside the technology rather than being designed into it.

We will take it.

Marcus—The Early Adopter Who Did Not Know What He Was Doing

Marcus Chen bought his first pair of Meta Ray-Ban Smart Glasses on a Tuesday in October because he had read the product review in *The Verge* and thought the open-ear audio sounded useful for morning calls. He is not, in his own self-description, a health-focused person. He is a product person—thirty-seven years old, VP of product at a Series B technology company in Austin, a competitive trail runner on weekends, the kind of person who owns five productivity apps and has read every issue of every newsletter about doing more with less. Health is something he manages. Performance is something he optimizes.

The glasses arrived on Thursday. By Friday morning he had restructured his first two hours around them. He took his 7:15 standup meeting walking—twenty minutes around his neighborhood, head level, eyes forward, processing overnight messages through the glasses while he moved. He answered two voice messages on the way back. He got to his desk at 8:15 feeling, as he put it to his wife that evening, "like I had already been awake for three hours but in a good way." He assumed it was the walk.

Six months later, Marcus also owns the Meta Oakley HSTN smart glasses—the athletic version, polarized, designed for trail running and cycling—and has restructured how he trains. He gets pace, elevation, and heart rate data through audio during runs. He navigates trails without once dropping his chin to a wrist or pulling out a phone. His trail pace has improved by eleven seconds per mile over six months. His HRV, tracked on an Oura ring, has risen seventeen points over the same period—which he cannot fully explain. His wife has mentioned, twice, that he seems less wired when he gets home. He has no framework for any of this. He simply knows something shifted around month three and has not shifted back.

Here is what Marcus has been doing physiologically, without knowing it. For the two to three hours per day he uses his glasses instead of his phone, his cervical spine carries ten to twelve pounds rather than sixty. His diaphragm has full room to descend. His visual field is forward-facing and wide—the panoramic mode that shifts the nervous system toward parasympathetic activity and the broad cognitive mode associated with creative and strategic thinking. He has been practicing the Twenty-Second Lift continuously for hours at a time, without once thinking of it as a practice. He thought he was answering emails more efficiently. He was restoring his nervous system.

Maya needs to understand the mechanism to practice the Lift deliberately. Marcus gets a fraction of the same benefit automatically, as a by-product of a technology choice made for entirely other reasons. This book gives Marcus what his glasses cannot: the understanding of why what is happening to him is happening. Once he has that understanding, he will not stop at two hours a day. He will restructure everything he can around the orientation that is already working—and he will understand, for the first time, exactly what he chooses when he picks up his phone instead of his glasses.

What Good Heads-Up Computing Should Do: Design Principles for the Next Generation

A book about the physiological consequences of computing interface design should be specific about what the next generation of devices should optimize. We offer the following design principles not as a complete specification, but as a starting framework for any product team building toward the heads-up future. These principles are derived from the physiology described throughout this book and from the clinical observations of three practitioners who have spent more than sixty combined years observing what computing interface design has done to the human nervous system.

Principle 1: Default Posture Should Be Heads-Up

The interface should be designed assuming the user's head is balanced over the spine and their gaze is directed forward at the horizon. Any feature that requires the user to look down or to compress their cervical spine to access it is a regression to the heads-down paradigm and should be designed out wherever possible. The first question of any product review should be: What does the user's head do during the typical use of this feature? If the answer is "drops forward," the design is incomplete.

Principle 2: Information Density Should Match Human Visual Capacity

The visual field has a foveal center (the eye's small zone of sharp central focus) capable of high-resolution processing and a peripheral surround designed for movement and contextual awareness. Heads-up interfaces that crowd the foveal center with high-density information replicate the cognitive narrowing of the smartphone era in a new form factor. Better interfaces use the peripheral field for ambient information and reserve the foveal center for the small percentage of moments that require focused attention. This is not only a comfort consideration. It is a nervous-system consideration: The panoramic visual mode is associated with parasympathetic activity and broad cognitive processing, while the narrow visual mode is associated with sympathetic activation and tunnel cognition.

Principle 3: Voice and Ambient Interaction Should Be the Default

Hand-and-eye interaction with a small visual target is the cervical-loading pattern of the smartphone era. Voice interaction is the natural inversion: It allows the user to keep their head balanced, their gaze open, and their hands free for the physical environment around them. The Meta Ray-Ban Smart Glasses demonstrated that voice-first consumer interaction can ship at scale and that users will adopt it. Future devices should treat voice as the default interaction modality and visual interaction as the exception, not the reverse.

Principle 4: The Device Should Read the Body, Not Only the Behavior

Engagement metrics—time on device, content consumed, actions taken—are the inheritance of the smartphone era and the proximate cause of the design choices that produced Tech Posture Syndrome. The next generation of devices must have the technical capacity to read the body itself: posture, breath, heartrate variability, gaze stability, autonomic state. A device that knows when its user has been in sustained sympathetic activation for two hours and gently adjusts its information-delivery accordingly is a device that has begun to take responsibility for its own physiological footprint. Build that.

Principle 5: The Interface Should Recommend Rest

No current consumer technology product, to our knowledge, is designed to recommend that its user disengage from it. This is the deepest pathology of the engagement-economy model: The product is incentivized against the user's well-being in the most fundamental way. The next generation of devices has the opportunity to invert this. A heads-up computing platform that, on detecting sustained physiological stress, suggests a five-minute walk, a breath practice, a moment of looking out at the horizon—and that measures its own success in part on the basis of the user's long-term physiological state rather than only by engagement minutes—is a product that has internalized a different definition of what success means. The companies that build this kind of product first will define the wellness-technology category for the decade that follows.

Principle 6: Children's Devices Require a Different Standard

The developmental nervous system of a child cannot be designed for using the same heuristics as the adult nervous system. Devices intended for use by children—including educational tablets, gaming devices, and any heads-up computing device marketed to families—should be designed under a higher standard that treats developmental physiology as a first-order constraint. This includes hard limits on sustained close-range visual focus, mandatory periods of far-distance visual engagement, postural variety requirements, and conservative defaults on engagement-maximizing features. The technology industry has the capacity to adopt these standards voluntarily. We hope it will. The alternative is regulatory imposition that will be cruder, slower, and less responsive to the specific physiological evidence than industry self-organization would be.

Principle 7: The Data Belongs to the Body It Came From

Biometric data collected by a wearable or a heads-up computing device is the most intimate data category any company has ever held. The principle that should govern its use is that the data exists to serve the human being it came from, not the company that collected it, not the advertisers it might be sold to, not the algorithms that might be trained on it without consent. Companies that internalize this principle and build their data architectures around it will earn the trust that the next generation of products requires. Companies that do not will be on the defensive, eventually and rightly, against regulatory and reputational consequences they could have avoided by getting the foundation right.

A Note on Implementation

We are aware that these principles are easier to articulate than to ship. Product organizations operate under commercial constraints, competitive pressures, engineering tradeoffs, and timeline realities that no outside framework can fully account for. We offer these principles in the spirit of partnership, not prescription. The companies building the heads-up future know their constraints better than we do. What we know is the physiology of the human bodies their products will engage. The collaboration between those two knowledge bases is the work the rest of this decade requires.

The Attention Economy Is Not New—And Policy Is Not Enough

Before we go further, a clear-eyed accounting of the current public conversation about technology and health is necessary—because this book exists inside that conversation and needs to be honest about where it agrees, where it adds nuance, and where it parts ways with the most prominent voices currently making the case for change.

Jonathan Haidt, the social psychologist whose book *The Anxious Generation* has become the most widely cited text on smartphone harms to adolescents, has documented with considerable rigor the correlation between smartphone adoption around 2012 and the subsequent decline in adolescent mental health—particularly among girls. His four-point prescription is institutional: no smartphones before high school, no social media before sixteen, phone-free schools, and more unsupervised play.

Tristan Harris, former Google design ethicist and cofounder of the Center for Humane Technology, has documented the deliberate design of engagement-maximizing features—infinite scroll, notification architecture, algorithmic amplification—and argued that these features are causing measurable harm to individuals and to democratic society. His prescription is also institutional: platform redesign, regulatory change, and new accountability structures.

Both men are serious, credible, and doing genuinely important work. We and the contents of this book agree with their diagnosis of the problem. We part ways—not in opposition but in scope—on the nature of the solution.

Here is the first thing worth naming clearly: The profit motive driving attention capture is not a new invention and treating it as one misidentifies the nature of the problem. Television was engineered to hold attention from its first decade. Radio competed for ears before that. The newspaper industry competed for eyeballs in the nineteenth century. Hollywood has spent a hundred years in the business of capturing human attention for two hours at a time and monetizing that capture through advertising. Madison Avenue has been the funding mechanism of mass media for over a century—and advertising's entire logic is that attention is the asset being bought and sold.

Every magazine on every newsstand, every billboard on every highway, every commercial between every television segment, is competing for the same resource that social media platforms compete for. The attention economy is the oldest business model in mass media. Treating it as a novel and uniquely alarming feature of the current moment produces a diagnosis that misses the specific thing that is new.

What is genuinely new is not the profit motive. It is two things: the speed of the feedback loop and the depth of the personalization. The algorithm updates in real time based on your individual behavior, not demographic averages. Your feed is optimized for you specifically—for the precise pattern of your engagement, your dwell time, your return frequency—in ways that no previous medium has been capable of. A television network programmed for a demographic. The algorithm programs for a person. That specificity, combined with the feedback loop speed that updates continuously, is the genuine novelty. It deserves serious attention. It does not require treating the profit motive as uniquely sinister when every media business in history has been organized around the same motive.

The second thing worth examining carefully is the institutional solution. Haidt and Harris are right that platform design and regulatory frameworks matter. They are also right that children, whose nervous systems and decision-making capacities are still being built, deserve specific protections that the adult autonomy framework does not fully provide. On this subject, the book is in agreement. Developmental windows are real. A thirteen-year-old cannot make the same fully informed choices about neurological inputs during peak plasticity that a forty-year-old can make about their own established nervous system.

But for adults—the primary audience of this book—the institutional solution has a timeline measured in decades, a track record of missing the nuance it is trying to protect, and a fundamental question it cannot answer: Who decides? If not the platforms, then governments. If not governments, then regulatory bodies. Each of these entities brings its own interests, blind spots, and capture risks. The food regulation parallel is exact: We have government agencies whose mandate is to determine what is safe and effective so that the public can make informed choices—not to make those choices for the public. The most we can ask of institutions is accurate information and honest labeling. The choice of what to consume, and how much, and when—that is the individual's decision. In a free society, it cannot be otherwise.

The timeline for policy solutions to technology harms is measured in decades. The timeline for personal change is measured in seconds. The most radical act available in the current technological environment is not lobbying for platform regulation. It is picking up the steering wheel.

The Accidental Redemption

There is a narrative arc in the story of Meta's technology that is worth naming directly, because it is one of the most consequential and least-discussed storylines in the history of the internet.

In 2004, Mark Zuckerberg launched Facebook from a dorm room at Harvard. In the years that followed, the company—through its own platforms and the broader social media ecosystem it helped create—became one of the primary architects of the Heads-Down World. The infinite scroll. The notification architecture. The engagement-maximizing algorithm that serves content calibrated for the physiological state of sympathetic activation. The product decisions that placed a close-range, forward-tilting screen in the hands of billions of people, including hundreds of millions of children during their most neurologically plastic years. These were not malicious decisions. They were commercial ones, made within a design frame that never included the human body in its field of consideration. The harm is real. The intent was elsewhere.

In 2023, Meta shipped the Ray-Ban Smart Glasses at consumer scale. In 2024, the Oakley HSTN collaboration brought the same technology into the athletic market. These products do not carry a single line of marketing language about cervical load, nervous system regulation, or the physiological consequences of sustained forward head posture. They are sold as convenience devices, fashion accessories, and performance tools for athletes. The companies that built them are motivated by the commercial logic of owning the next computing platform—not by any recognition of what the previous platform did to the bodies of the people who adopted it.

And yet, the outcome of that commercial bet—if it reaches the scale Meta intends, if it is equipped with the biometric sensing and AI coaching that the technology road map points toward, if it does for billions of people what it has inadvertently done for Marcus—is genuinely redemptive. Not because the company intended redemption. Because the trajectory of their commercial vision happens to align with the physiological needs of the species they disrupted. The same company whose early products helped create the Heads-Down World has made the largest single corporate investment in the technology that could end it.

History does not require intent to deliver justice. The steam engine was not built to give working people mobility—but it did. The internet was not built to democratize knowledge—but it did. Meta's heads-up computing platform was not built to heal the physiological harm of the smartphone era—but it might. The science in this book is the framework that makes that healing legible: the mechanism through which the harm occurred, the mechanism through which the reversal is available, and the specific product features that would make the reversal systematic rather than accidental.

Whether Meta reads this book and builds what chapter 13 describes is beyond our knowledge. But the invitation is here, in these pages, for any engineer, any product manager, any executive at any technology company who is willing to ask the question that was never asked when the smartphone was designed: What does this do to the human body? The answer is documented. The correction is available. The technology to deliver it at scale is closer than it has ever been.

> The company that created the Heads-Down World is building the technology that could end it. That is not redemption by design. It is redemption by trajectory—and it is available to any company willing to read the science, understand the mechanism, and build what the human nervous system actually needs from the devices it spends eleven hours a day with.

The Honest Caveat

The Generation That Grew Up Heads-Up

There is a dimension of the heads-up computing revolution that has received almost no discussion in the technology press or in the healthcare literature, but that may be its most consequential long-term implication: the children who grow up with heads-up computing as their primary interface will not experience the Heads-Down World.

A child who learns to read through glasses that bring the text to their eye level, rather than a tablet they hold below their face, is building their visual and postural architecture inside a different interface. A child who plays games that require them to look outward, to move through physical space, to engage their full proprioceptive system rather than their thumbs and their eyes alone, is developing their nervous system inside an experience that is closer to what the human nervous system evolved to receive than what the smartphone generation has received.

The developmental window argument from chapter 2 runs in the positive direction as well as the negative. The windows that are vulnerable to the harm of heads-down technology are also available to the benefit of heads-up technology. A child who spends the sensitive period for visual development with an interface that exercises the full range of visual focal distances—near, middle, and far—is building visual processing capacity that the tablet generation has been denied. A child whose primary movement experiences include the full proprioceptive complexity of real-world navigation rather than sedentary close-range screen engagement is developing a nervous system calibrated to the full richness of physical experience.

This is the most hopeful projection available from the heads-up computing trajectory: not merely that adults will be less damaged by their technology, but that children who grow up inside a heads-up interface will not need to be restored to a physiological baseline they never lost. The Look Up Practice is, at its deepest level, a restoration practice—returning the body to inputs it was designed to receive but has been denied. The generation that grows up with those inputs as the baseline of their technological experience will not need to restore what they never lost.

They will simply look up. Because that is what their technology always asked of them. And the nervous systems they build inside that experience will be the inheritance they bring to every problem the world will need them to solve.

Heads-up computing addresses the postural problem. It does not automatically solve everything.

You Are the Driver

Here is the most important reframe available to anyone who is serious about their relationship with technology: You are not a passenger. You are the driver.

Think about what it means to drive a car. You put your hands on the steering wheel because steering is your responsibility. The road does not choose your destination. The weather does not choose your speed. The other cars do not choose your lane. You do. And the quality of your driving—the precision of your steering, your appropriate speed for conditions, your willingness to pull over when you need to rest—depends on the state of the person behind the wheel. A tired driver drifts. An impaired driver overcorrects. A regulated, alert driver navigates competently through conditions that would overwhelm a compromised one.

Your attention works the same way. The platform is the road. The algorithm is the weather. The content is the landscape you are moving through. None of these are driving the car. You are. And the quality of your navigation depends entirely on the physiological state of the nervous system doing the navigating.

This is where the dysregulation argument becomes most precise and most personal. The person scrolling in sympathetic activation—chest compressed, breath shallow, nervous system running slightly hot from hours of sustained postural load—is not driving well. They are drifting. The activating content captures their dwell time not because they consciously chose it but because the threat-activated nervous system is literally more sensitive to threat stimuli. The algorithm reads the dwell time as preference and serves more. The driver did not choose this destination. Their physiological state steered them there while they were not paying attention.

Gary Vaynerchuk—an entrepreneur and one of the most thoughtful voices on the actual mechanics of social media engagement—makes an argument worth taking seriously: The feed reflects the user, not the other way around. Search for rainbows and ponies and watch what your feed shows you within twenty-four hours. The algorithm responds to what you engage with. If you do not like where your feed is taking you, the first question is not what the platform is doing wrong. The first question should be what you have been steering toward.

This book extends that argument further than Vaynerchuk takes it. The feed reflects not only your conscious choices but also your physiological state. A person in chronic sympathetic activation, scrolling through the landscape of the internet, generates engagement signals that are different from the engagement signals of a person in the ventral vagal state—regulated, open, curious rather than threatened. The algorithm cannot distinguish between conscious preference and physiological reactivity.

It sees dwell time. It serves more of what generates dwell time. The regulated nervous system, which dwells differently, generates different signals and receives a different feed. You are not only what you consciously choose to engage with. You are the physiological state you bring to the engagement. Change the state—with twenty seconds, before you open the app—and you change the driver. Change the driver and you change where the car goes.

The same principle governs scrolling speed. Scrolling slowly is a physiological act. The regulated nervous system naturally decelerates—it makes real contact with content rather than skimming the surface, notices what it is doing in response to what it is seeing and retains the capacity to steer away from what is not serving it. The dysregulated nervous system races. It consumes content without tasting. It drifts toward the most activating content because activation is the state it is already in, and activation is self-reinforcing. The practice of slowing down is not a discipline you impose on yourself from outside. It is the natural behavior of a nervous system that is driving rather than being driven.

And pulling over—the voluntary choice to put the phone down, to close the app, to step out of the vehicle and look at the actual world—is the most important driving skill available. Not stopping at a red light that an external authority forces on you. The internal recognition that you need to rest, that the road you have been on is not taking you where you want to go, that the most useful thing you can do right now is to be somewhere other than inside the feed. This is PAIN applied to technology: Pay attention inside now. Notice what your nervous system is doing in response to what you are consuming. Make the adult decision to steer toward something better.

> Nobody is forcing you to look at your phone for eleven hours a day. The phone is not attached to your face. The scroll does not continue without your thumb. The notification can be turned off. The app can be deleted. These are choices—choices that are influenced by design and habit and physiological state, but choices, nonetheless. The most empowering truth available to anyone reading this book is that they are already holding the steering wheel. They have been holding it all along. PAIN is the instrument panel. The Twenty-Second Lift is the recalibration. Looking up is the choice to drive well.

What Technology Has Actually Given Us

There is a dimension of the current conversation about technology and health that is almost never named in the way it deserves to be named, and its absence makes the conversation less honest and less useful. So let us name it directly.

We are living inside the most astonishing expansion of human connection, knowledge access, and creative possibility in the history of our species. A person living just a century ago had access to the knowledge and social connection available within a radius of perhaps fifty miles. A person almost anywhere today has in their pocket the accumulated knowledge of human civilization, real-time connection with any other human being on earth, the creative output of every artist and musician and writer alive, the ability to build a business, find a community, learn a skill, access a medical diagnosis, translate a language, navigate an unknown city, or connect with someone who shares their most obscure passion—from anywhere, instantly, for free.

This is not a small thing. It is one of the most consequential gifts any generation has ever received. The smartphone did not only take, it gave. It continues to give, every day, to billions of people whose lives are materially better because of what it made possible. The researcher in Lagos who can access every journal ever published. The small business owner in rural Kentucky who can reach a global customer. The teenager in a small town who finds, online, the community that confirms they are not alone in who they are. The grandmother who sees her grandchild's face on a screen every Sunday morning. These are real gifts. They deserve to be named with the same seriousness that the harms deserve to be named.

The argument of this book is not that the technology is bad. It is that most people are engaging with extraordinary technology in a physiological state that prevents them from receiving its full gift and makes them susceptible to its worst costs. The solution is not to get out of the car. Cars are extraordinary. They have transformed human life. The solution is to drive well. To bring the regulated, alert, physiologically resourced nervous system to the wheel. To choose speed and destination deliberately. To notice when you are drifting and correct. To pull over and rest when you need to.

The technology is extraordinary. You are the driver. PAIN is the instrument panel. The rest is navigation.

The person spending eight hours per day in AR glasses—however perfectly heads-up their posture—is still spending eight hours in sustained computational engagement. The attentional fragmentation, the reduced face-to-face contact, the challenge of genuine recovery: These remain. The practices in this book are not made obsolete by better technology. They are made more effective because the physiological starting point is better.

Better interface design and better personal physiological practice are partners in the future, not alternatives to each other. The Heads-Down World created the problem at civilization scale. Heads-up computing can resolve it at a civilizational scale. The practices in this book are the bridge between where we are and where that future arrives.

Key Takeaways:

- The problem is the interface, not the technology—heads-down computing required the human body to adapt to the machine; heads-up computing inverts this.
- Eleven billion human hours per day of forward head posture is a civilizational health problem requiring structural as well as individual solutions.
- Heads-up computing is the first computing paradigm in history to treat human biology as a primary design constraint.
- Meta's AR commitment, alongside Apple's and Google's parallel investments, signals that the largest technology organizations in the world are collectively betting on a heads-up future.
- The practices in this book are the bridge—they address the physiological damage of the current interface while the future arrives, and they remain essential even after it does.

Put It into Practice

Spend thirty minutes today using only heads-up computing: voice commands for tasks you would normally perform on your phone, with your device put away and your head in a neutral, forward position. Notice your posture, your breath, your visual field during those thirty minutes. Notice the quality of your attention and the state of your body. That experience is a small preview of the direction the entire interface is moving. You can begin living there, in small increments, right now.

CHAPTER 13

AI, Augmented Reality, and the Future of Human Vitality

The Feedback Loop That Changes Everything

The most powerful technology will not just measure your vitality.
It will help you build it.

Maya has been tracking her sleep on her phone for three years. She looks at the number each morning—seven hours, six and a half, sometimes five—and does not know what to do with it beyond feeling better or worse about the night she had.

This is what most wearable technology looks like for most people: a number, delivered daily, that sits between the person and any meaningful change they might make because of it. The gap between having the data and knowing what to do with it is the gap this chapter reveals. And closing the gap requires understanding something most people have never been told: that not all wearable technology is the same kind of thing.

> There are wearables that report your biology. And there are wearables that support it. These are not the same tool. They are not even in the same category. Knowing which you have—and what to do with each—may be the most practically important distinction in this entire chapter.

Two Categories of Technology—Only One Changes Anything

The first category is biometric tracking technology. This is what most people mean when they talk about wearables. A device—a watch, a ring, a clip—that measures physiological activity and reports it back to you as data. Steps. Heart rate. Sleep score. Calories. HRV. The device observes. It records. It displays.

Think of it as the rearview mirror of your health. It shows you what already happened. You slept badly. You moved less than yesterday. Your HRV dropped on Wednesday. The information is real. The problem is that the mirror offers no steering wheel. It reports on the road you have already driven. It does not help you navigate what is coming.

The second category is functional support technology. This is categorically different, and most people do not yet know it exists. A functional support device does not simply observe and report. It detects a shift in your physiological state and delivers an intervention before the downstream consequences accumulate. It does not wait for you to check your data. It meets you in the moment when the moment matters.

Several devices in this category are available to consumers right now, today. The Apollo Neuro wearable delivers gentle vibration patterns that the nervous system reads as a safety signal—measurably shifting the autonomic balance toward parasympathetic dominance within minutes of use. The Sensate device uses infrasound vibration applied to the sternum to stimulate the vagus nerve directly, producing documented improvements in HRV and self-reported stress. The HeartMath Inner Balance sensor pairs with a smartphone app to train cardiac coherence—the resonant breathing pattern at six breaths per minute described in chapter 7—using real-time biofeedback to guide the user toward and sustain the target state.

These devices are not mentioned here as endorsements. They are mentioned because they represent, concretely, what functional support technology looks like in its current form—and because most people who would benefit from them have never heard of them, because they have no category for what they are. They are not fitness trackers. They are not medical devices. They are nervous system support tools. The category does not yet have a name that everyone knows. That will change. For now, the important thing is that you know the distinction exists—and that you can seek out the category deliberately rather than assuming that any wearable that collects data about your body is also doing something useful with it.

The distinction is not subtle. A rearview mirror and a navigation system both involve information about position. But one shows you where you were and the other changes where you are going. Biometric tracking and functional support both involve data about your body. But one records your history and the other shapes your future.

Why the Nervous System Is the Right Target

The nervous system is upstream from every other system in the body. Cardiovascular function, immune response, hormonal balance, cognitive performance, mood regulation, sleep architecture—all of these are downstream outputs of nervous system state. Which means that a wearable that intervenes at the level of the nervous system is intervening at the point of maximum leverage. It is addressing the coordinator of everything else, rather than any single downstream metric.

A step counter addresses one downstream metric. A sleep tracker addresses another. A calorie monitor addresses a third. Each is useful within its domain. None of them touches the system that regulates all of the domains simultaneously.

This is the strategic case for nervous-system-centered wearables: not that they are better than other trackers at measuring what other trackers measure, but that they are operating at a different level of the hierarchy entirely. Maximum impact. Minimum effort. Upstream from everything else.

If You Only Have a Tracker: How to Give the Data Meaning

Most people reading this book have a tracking device, not a functional support device. That is fine. Tracking data is genuinely valuable—when you know how to use it. The problem is not the data. The problem is the absence of a framework for interpretation. Here is one.

Stop reading the number. Start reading the pattern.

A single night's HRV score is almost meaningless in isolation. Your HRV trend across thirty days—rising, falling, stable, or volatile—is a signal about the direction of your nervous system's regulatory capacity. That direction is the thing to track. Not the number. The direction.

Ask three questions of your data every week, not every morning.

- **First:** What was my physiological state at its best this week, and what preceded it?
- **Second:** What was it at its lowest, and what preceded that?
- **Third:** What practice, if any, correlated with the better outcomes?

These three questions transform tracking data from a scorecard into a feedback loop. A scorecard tells you how you did. A feedback loop tells you what to do differently.

Maya has three years of sleep data. She has never asked those three questions. She has been keeping score. If she starts keeping a feedback loop instead, that same data—the same numbers, the same device, no additional purchase required—becomes a map of her own nervous system patterns. The tool did not change. The framework changed. And the framework is everything.

This distinction—between tracking compliance with normal ranges and building genuine physiological self-literacy—is worth dwelling on, because it marks the precise point where the medical monitoring model and the Look Up model part ways.

The medical remote monitoring infrastructure being built right now by health systems worldwide shares the hardware—wearables, sensors, continuous tracking—with the functional support technology described earlier in this chapter. But it operates from a completely different framework. The medical model asks: Is this person's reading outside the normal range? If yes, trigger an alert. If the alert is confirmed, trigger a protocol. The protocol almost always involves a pharmaceutical intervention designed to bring the reading back within range.

Notice what this model does not ask. It does not ask:

- Is this person thriving?
- Is their nervous system expressing its full regulatory capacity?
- Are they growing, adapting, present, vital?
- Is the quality of their attention, their resilience, their presence in their relationships moving in a positive direction?

These questions have no instrument in the medical monitoring model. A person with perfectly compliant blood pressure, normal HRV, and within-range glucose readings may be experiencing exactly what Maya experiences—and the entire algorithmic infrastructure will report: "No intervention required."

The framework in this book asks a different question of the same data. Not: Am I within range? But: Am I moving toward my best possible function? Not: Is an intervention required? But: What input does my nervous system need right now—what whisper is it sending that I can respond to before it becomes a scream? The technology is the same. The orientation is completely different. One produces compliance. The other produces vitality. And only one of them requires you to pay attention inside now.

The Behavior Change Problem

The fundamental challenge of behavior change is not knowledge. Most people who read this book will understand, by the time they reach this chapter, precisely what the Twenty-Second Lift involves and why it works. The challenge is doing it consistently—across the full complexity and variability of daily life, for long enough that it becomes habitual rather than effortful.

The Arithmetic of a Different Direction

Let us be specific about what the compound interest of physiological practice actually looks like, because the abstraction—small inputs, large returns, the magic of consistency—can obscure the concrete reality that makes it worth taking seriously.

A person who adds the Twenty-Second Lift to every phone pickup—a conservative average of thirty times per day—performs six hundred seconds of deliberate physiological recalibration daily. That is ten minutes. Distributed across a day in twenty-second intervals, attached to existing triggers, requiring no scheduled time and no separate motivation. Ten minutes of upstream nervous system intervention, compounded across a year, is sixty hours. Sixty hours of deliberate physiological input, distributed in the way the research on autonomic regulation suggests, is most effective: frequent brief interventions rather than occasional long ones.

What do sixty hours of upstream nervous system intervention compound to? The research on HRV trends offers the clearest answer. Studies following individuals through consistent stress-reduction and physiological practice protocols consistently find that HRV—the most sensitive measure of nervous system regulatory capacity—improves measurably over periods of eight to twelve weeks of consistent practice and continues to improve across years of sustained practice. The nervous system does not plateau the way a muscle does. Its regulatory capacity deepens across time in ways that correlate with every health outcome we care about: cardiovascular function, immune resilience, cognitive performance, emotional regulation, sleep quality, and longevity.

The person who has practiced the Look Up Practice for five years is not five times better than the person who has practiced it for one year. They are categorically different in their physiological baseline. The nervous system that has been consistently supported for five years is a more capable system—more adaptive, more resilient, more able to sustain performance under load and recover from challenge—than the same nervous system would have been without that support. This is not a promise. It is the well-documented outcome of consistent upstream physiological investment, drawn from decades of research in autonomic neuroscience, exercise physiology, and mind-body medicine.

Maya, at thirty-eight, has somewhere between forty and fifty years of working and relational life ahead of her. Every year of her life that her nervous system spends trending toward its best regulatory capacity is a year that builds on the year before. The compound return on starting now—not in the best possible circumstances, not with the full protocol executed perfectly, but with the imperfect, consistent, trigger-paired twenty-second practice that is the minimum effective dose—is incalculable in the way that all genuinely compound returns are incalculable from any individual input.

The most important financial decision anyone makes is when to start investing. The same principle governs physiological investment. The best time to begin was when the Heads-Down World began, before the accumulation had built up. The second-best time is now.

AI coaching addresses this challenge directly. Not by providing more information—the information is already here—but by providing the right intervention at the right moment with increasing personalization over time.

What AI Coaching Can Do

- **Continuous biometric monitoring:** Wearable devices tracking heart rate variability, respiratory rate, movement patterns, and postural indicators provide a continuous stream of physiological data. AI systems can interpret this data in real time and deliver feedback calibrated to the individual's current state—not generic scheduled reminders, but interventions timed to the moments of maximum physiological relevance.
- **Personalized pattern recognition:** AI systems can identify each user's specific vulnerability patterns—the time of day when HRV drops most reliably, the activities that most consistently precede state deterioration, the practices that produce the greatest individual response—and use these patterns to continuously improve the precision of its guidance.
- **Adaptive progression:** Interventions calibrated to the individual's current capacity produce superior adherence compared to fixed standards. AI coaching modulates the intensity and complexity of practices as the user's capacity evolves, creating a system that grows with the person.
- **Longitudinal insight:** AI systems can identify trends invisible to the person in the middle of their own experience—the seasonal patterns, the workload correlations, the relationship between specific practices and specific outcomes measured weeks later.

The Signals That Matter and the Interventions They Should Trigger

Existing wearable devices collect a remarkable volume of physiological data. The challenge is not measurement. The challenge is converting measurement into the right intervention at the right moment. The framework that follows maps the signals current wearables can already detect to the specific physiological interventions this book has been describing. It is offered as a working document for any product team building the AI-coaching layer of the heads-up future.

Signal: Sustained Elevated Resting Heart Rate Without Activity Context

What it indicates: Sympathetic activation in the absence of physical demand. The user is in stress physiology while sitting at a desk.
Recommended intervention: A gentle, nondisruptive prompt to engage in three breath cycles with extended exhale (four counts in, eight counts out). The intervention takes thirty to ninety seconds. Heart rate variability begins shifting within the first cycle. The prompt is delivered through ambient audio if the user is wearing heads-up audio, or through a low-priority haptic if they are wearing only a wrist device.
What to measure: Heart rate trajectory in the five minutes following the intervention. If the intervention reliably correlates with downward heart rate trajectory in this user, the system increases prompt frequency for similar future contexts. If it does not, the system tries an alternate intervention.

Signal: Heart Rate Variability Trending Below Personal Baseline Across Multiple Days

What it indicates: Cumulative nervous-system regulatory load—the user has been in sustained dysregulation for long enough that single-intervention responses are insufficient.
Recommended intervention: A weekly pattern-review prompt that surfaces what has changed in the user's recent context (sleep, schedule density, exercise, social engagement) and offers a small structural change recommendation rather than a moment-of-stress intervention. Examples: "Your HRV has been declining for nine days. The strongest correlation in your data is reduced morning movement. Adding a ten-minute walk before screens would likely reverse the trend within a week."
What to measure: Whether the user accepts the structural recommendation, whether they implement it, and whether the HRV trend reverses. The system's personalization improves through these feedback loops over months.

Signal: Forward Head Posture Detected Through Glasses-Mounted Inertial Sensors or Companion Device

What it indicates: The user has slipped from heads-up orientation into heads-down orientation, accumulating cervical load and compressing the diaphragm.

Recommended intervention: Brief peripheral visual cue (in the case of AR-capable devices) or low-priority haptic (in the case of wrist-only devices) prompting the Twenty-Second Lift. Cue should be calibrated to the minimum intensity that produces user response without becoming an annoyance—and should be silenced after a single ignore.
What to measure: Postural recovery within sixty seconds of the prompt. Frequency of successful interventions per day. Long-term postural baseline trajectory across weeks.

Signal: Sleep Architecture Disruption—Reduced Deep Sleep, Fragmented REM, Elevated Sleeping Heart Rate

What it indicates: Nervous system has not transitioned to parasympathetic dominance overnight, often correlated with evening screen exposure, late food, or sustained daytime sympathetic load.
Recommended intervention: Morning surfacing of the previous evening's pattern in the user's evening alignment routine, with a single small change recommendation focused on the most modifiable upstream variable. Avoid the temptation to overwhelm with diagnostic complexity—the AI coaching layer's value is in selecting the single highest-leverage adjustment for this user in this week, not in providing comprehensive analysis.
What to measure: Whether the recommended adjustment is implemented and whether sleep architecture improves in the subsequent week.

Signal: Voice Stress Markers in User Communications

What it indicates: Acute sympathetic activation in the moment, often during or following difficult conversations or stressful work content.
Recommended intervention: Post-event prompt for the threshold practice—twenty seconds of physiological recovery before the next context begins. Particularly valuable in transition moments between work blocks, between meetings, or before relational engagements.
What to measure: User-reported quality of the subsequent interaction, when the user opts to provide it. Long-term improvement in voice stress baseline across months of consistent threshold-practice usage.

A Note on Aggregation and Restraint

A coaching system that prompts users at every detectable deviation from baseline becomes an annoyance in days and an ignored notification in weeks. The discipline of an effective AI coaching layer is restraint—surfacing only the interventions that matter most, in the moments most likely to be acted on, at frequencies that the user's relationship with the device can sustain over years rather than weeks. The right metric for the coaching layer is not engagement with the prompts. It is the long-term physiological trajectory of the user. Build to that metric.

The AR Coaching Layer

When AI coaching integrates with augmented reality interfaces, the possibilities expand significantly. Your AR glasses detect, through built-in biometric sensors and postural analysis, that your head has migrated forward by two inches and your HRV has dropped below your personal threshold. A gentle visual cue appears at the periphery of your visual field. You pause, do the Twenty-Second Lift, and the system logs the response: Your HRV begins recovering within forty-five seconds.

Over months, the system develops a model of your physiology more precise than any standardized recommendation. It knows when your body needs what particular input. It offers that input at the moment of maximum relevance, in the form most likely to be acted on—without requiring you to remember, schedule, or motivate yourself.

This is not surveillance. This is support—the physiological equivalent of a skilled practitioner who knows your patterns and knows exactly when to intervene.

The Destination: Physiological Self-Literacy

The goal of AI coaching is not permanent dependence on a system. It is the development, through the system's scaffolding, of genuine physiological self-literacy.

Maya has been collecting sleep data for three years. Imagine instead that she had spent three years with a system that showed her: Your HRV drops on the evenings when you don't do the evening alignment. Your afternoon cognitive performance is measurably higher on the days when you take a ten-minute walk at noon. Your anxiety scores on the weeks when you skip the morning alignment are 20 percent higher than your baseline.

After three years of that feedback, Maya would not need the system to tell her what to do. She would know—in the deeply personal, physiologically grounded way that changes behavior permanently—what her body requires and what happens when it doesn't receive it. The scaffolding is no longer needed because the self-literacy it built has become her own.

> The future is not technology replacing human self-knowledge. It is technology accelerating the development of it—so that the understanding Dr. LaMarche arrived at through a terminal diagnosis, most people can arrive at through a wearable and a year of attention.

From Rearview Mirror to Health GPS

The single most useful frame for understanding what the next generation of biometric technology needs to become is the difference between a rearview mirror and a GPS navigation system. Both look at the same road. They serve completely different functions.

A rearview mirror tells you where you have been. It is useful for a specific purpose—confirming you are not about to be hit from behind—but it does not tell you where to go, when to turn, or how to reach your destination. The current generation of wearable health devices, despite their extraordinary measurement capabilities, are mostly rearview mirrors. They show you what your body did yesterday. They generate scores. They alert you when a number falls outside a range. They are scorecards, retrospective and reactive, with no inherent capacity to tell you what to do next.

A GPS navigation system is the opposite. It knows where you are. It knows where you are trying to go. It plots the route. It replans in real time when conditions change. It tells you when to turn, what to expect, and how long until you arrive. It does not require you to interpret data and figure out what to do with it. It tells you what to do, in real time, with confidence calibrated to the actual situation.

The biometric devices of the next decade should be health GPS systems, not rearview mirrors. They should know your physiological starting point. They should know where you are trying to go—better sleep, more energy, sustained focus, deeper recovery, longer health span. They should plot the daily route from where you are to where you are heading. They should tell you, in real time, what to do next: This is the moment to take a walk, this is the moment to do the Twenty-Second Lift, this is the night to prioritize sleep over the meeting that could be moved, this is the week to schedule a Tune-In and Tune-Up with your Human Doctor.

The transition from rearview mirror to GPS is not primarily a hardware transition. The hardware exists. The transition is a framework transition—from data presentation to decision support, from compliance monitoring to vitality navigation, from "here is what your body did" to "here is what your body is asking for, right now." Companies that make this transition will define the wearable category for the decade that follows. Companies that do not will be selling rearview mirrors in a world that has moved to navigation.

Oura, with its sustained focus on HRV and sleep architecture, is closer to GPS than most. Whoop's recovery and strain framework points in the same direction. Apple Health's integration capabilities create the platform for it. Garmin's athletic performance ecosystem already operates as navigation rather than scorecard for the user populations it serves best. The convergence is underway. The framework in this book—the upstream variable of nervous system state, the specific interventions calibrated to physiological inputs, the directional question of "where are you trying to go"—is the missing layer that turns the convergence into a category-defining transition.

> You are not your data. You are the body the data came from. The devices of the next decade should be in the business of helping you become more fully alive—not in the business of grading the body you already are. That is the difference between rearview mirror and GPS. That is the transition this book is calling for.

The Future We Are Building—A Product Road Map for Human Vitality

The technology that would make Marcus's accidental discovery systematic—and would make Maya's deliberate practice effortless—does not yet fully exist. But every component required to build it either exists already or is in active development. What follows is not speculation. It is a product road map, derived from the science in this book, for the technology company that wants to lead the next decade of human health.

Postural detection in ambient computing. The camera array already built into Meta's Ray-Ban Smart Glasses could, with appropriate software, detect forward head posture in real time—not by measuring the user directly, but by analyzing the angle of their visual field relative to the horizon. When the gaze drops below a threshold for more than ninety seconds, a gentle tone through the open-ear speaker prompts the Lift. No screen. No vibration. No interruption of workflow. The user does not look at a device. The device reads the user's orientation and responds. Twenty seconds of intervention delivered invisibly, continuously, throughout the day—at the moment of maximum physiological relevance rather than at a scheduled time chosen in advance.

HRV-triggered breath guidance. The next generation of smart glasses with integrated PPG sensors—measuring pulse through the temporal artery at the temple where glasses naturally rest—could detect HRV in real time. When HRV drops below the user's personal threshold, the AI coaching layer delivers the physiological sigh through the open-ear speaker: a gentle prompt, two counts in through the nose, long exhale through the mouth. The user takes the breath.

HRV begins recovering within forty-five seconds. The system logs the response. Over months, it develops a model of the user's physiology more precise than any standardized recommendation. It knows when their nervous system needs what particular input. It offers that input in real time, at the moment of maximum relevance—not at a scheduled reminder time, but when the body is calling for it. This is proactive PAIN delivered at scale through a device the user is wearing anyway.

The Look Up Metric. A single composite score—derived from postural orientation data, HRV trend, respiratory rate, movement variety, and sleep quality—that answers the question the medical monitoring model has no instrument for: not "are your metrics in range?" but "are you becoming more fully alive?" The Look Up Metric is not a medical score. It does not diagnose. It measures the direction of vitality: whether the user is trending toward their best physiological expression or away from it. It answers, in a single number updated in real time, the question every human being is living with: not "How is my blood pressure?" but rather "How am I doing?"

Social vitality synchronization. Research has documented that two people in genuine attunement—face-to-face, nervous systems regulated, social engagement circuits fully active—show measurable convergence in their HRV patterns. A subtle peripheral indicator in the visual field of glasses worn by both participants in a high-stakes conversation could signal when that quality of connection has been achieved—and when it has been lost. Not as surveillance but a mirror for the thing human beings evolved to do with each other and have been losing the capacity for, one screen hour at a time. The most important meetings in any organization are not the ones with the best slides. They are the ones where the nervous systems in the room are sufficiently regulated to access the social intelligence that good decisions require. Technology that helps people find and sustain that state would be worth more than any presentation tool ever built.

The Human Doctor integration layer. The Human Doctor who has assessed a patient's postural pattern and HRV baseline can access, with patient consent, their longitudinal Look Up Metric data. They can see the correlation between spinal adjustment frequency and HRV trend; between the Twenty-Second Lift consistency and afternoon cognitive performance; between the morning alignment practice and sleep quality scores. They can see, in the data, what the patient cannot see from the inside of their own experience—the pattern across weeks and months that makes the clinical recommendation precise rather than generic. The Human Doctor is not replaced by the platform. The platform makes every in-person encounter more informed, more targeted, and more likely to produce the outcome both the practitioner and the patient are working toward.

These are not speculative features from a distant future. They are also the meeting point of the three intelligences—universal, innate, and artificial—that chapter 14 names directly. Each one is derivable from technology in current production—the camera arrays, the PPG sensors, the AI coaching architectures, the biometric data pipelines—applied to a framework that this book is the first to articulate in full.

The technology company that builds this stack will not be building a wellness product. It will be building the infrastructure for the second future described in chapter 10—the future in which technology serves vitality rather than merely surveilling pathology. That company will not need to choose between commercial success and human benefit. In this domain, at this particular moment in history, those two objectives are the same objective.

Key Takeaways:

- Two categories of wearable technology serve fundamentally different functions: biometric tracking (the rearview mirror—reporting what already happened) and functional support technology (real-time intervention in nervous system state). Knowing which you have, and how to use each, determines whether the technology changes anything.
- The nervous system is upstream from every other system in the body—cardiovascular, immune, hormonal, cognitive, and emotional. A wearable that intervenes at the nervous system level is therefore intervening at the point of maximum leverage with minimum effort, rather than addressing any single downstream metric.
- The integration of AI coaching with AR interfaces creates real-time, context-sensitive physiological support delivered in the user's field of view at moments of maximum relevance.
- If you only have a tracking device: Stop reading the daily number and start reading the weekly pattern. Ask these questions of your data each week: When was my state best, and what preceded it? When was it lowest, and what preceded that? What practice correlated with better outcomes? This converts a scorecard into a feedback loop.
- AI coaching closes the gap between tracking data and meaningful action—delivering the right intervention at the right moment with increasing personalization over time, addressing the behavior change problem that knowledge and tracking alone cannot solve.

Put It Into Practice

First: Identify which category of technology you are currently using.

Do your devices observe and report—or do they detect and intervene?

If you only have tracking devices, apply the three-question framework to your data this week:

- When was my physiological state highest and what preceded it?
- When was it lowest and what preceded that?
- What practice correlated with better outcomes?

Do not check the number every morning. Check the pattern every Sunday. One insight from that pattern—one genuine behavioral adjustment based on what you find—is worth more than a year of daily number-checking. That is the difference between a rearview mirror and a map. You already have the data. Begin using it as navigation.

PART IV
THE MOVEMENT

An Invitation to Live with Vitality

CHAPTER 14

The Three Intelligences

Universal, Innate, and Artificial

The subtitle of this book is *The New Science of Vitality in the Age of AI.* The word that has not yet been discussed at the depth it deserves is "intelligence." This chapter is about what the word means, where it comes from, and how the three intelligences operating in your life—Universal Intelligence, Innate Intelligence, and artificial intelligence—should be ordered if you want a life of coherence, vitality, and flourishing rather than one of confusion, depletion, and inversion.

A note before we begin. The chiropractic profession has been using the terms Universal Intelligence and Innate Intelligence for more than 130 years. The terms originate in D. D. Palmer's founding writings on chiropractic in the 1890s. We are chiropractors, and the heritage of these concepts is part of our clinical tradition. We believe those concepts are too important to be confined to the tradition that first named them, and we are writing this chapter for a broader audience than the profession alone.

We will use the words with their historical weight where that weight serves the argument. We will also open them up in language that stands on its own regardless of the reader's relationship to chiropractic, to any religious tradition, or to any particular metaphysical framework. Readers will bring different framings to these concepts. The argument we are making does not require any specific framing. It asks only that you consider what is true about the reality you are already living in.

Universal Intelligence

There is an organizing principle in the universe. Physicists call it the laws of physics. Biologists call it evolution by natural selection. Mathematicians call it the structure that makes mathematics possible. Chemists call it the periodic table. Theologians call it God. Philosophers call it the ground of being, or the logos, or simply order. Systems thinkers call it emergent self-organization.

Whatever you call it, something is organizing. Matter is not chaos. Energy does not distribute randomly. The universe has structure at every scale we can measure, from the subatomic to the cosmological, and that structure produces, over time, ordered complexity of a specific and lawful kind. Stars form. Planets form. Molecules assemble into living cells. Cells assemble into bodies. Bodies assemble into societies. Societies develop languages, sciences, and technologies that reveal still more of the underlying order. The organizing did not stop at any point. It continues. You are reading this book inside a universe that is still organizing, still producing more ordered complexity, still expressing whatever principle is behind the organization.

We will call that principle Universal Intelligence, because the term is as good as any other for pointing at it. You may substitute the name from your own tradition. What we mean by the term is not a theological claim about a personal deity, though readers who hold that framework will find nothing here that contradicts it. What we mean is the observable fact that the universe has an organizing structure, that the organizing structure produces ordered complexity rather than chaos, and that the ordered complexity includes the body you are reading this book with, the mind you are reading it through, and the capacity for attention that makes the reading meaningful.

These are not accidents. They are expressions of a universe with an organizing principle that is real, is operative, and is worth taking seriously as the context within which every other intelligence in your life is operating.

A life lived in alignment with Universal Intelligence is one kind of life. A life lived against it—fighting the body's design, ignoring its signals, overriding its capacities with suppression and intervention—is a very different kind of life. Most people in the Heads-Down World are living the second kind without knowing it. The first kind is available to them. It begins with acknowledging that the body they are inhabiting was not designed by them, was not engineered by the technology companies whose products they use, and is not optimizable through any combination of supplements, apps, or algorithms.

It was produced by a universe with an organizing principle that is older, deeper, and wiser than any human system can match. The appropriate response to that recognition is humility—not passivity, but humility—and a willingness to listen to what the body, as an expression of that larger intelligence, is telling you about how to live well inside it.

Innate Intelligence

Universal Intelligence is the larger order. Innate Intelligence is what that larger order looks like in the specific, local, individual form of your body.

Your body is, right now, performing operations of staggering complexity that you are not consciously managing. Your heart is beating. Your breath is cycling. Your immune system is patrolling for pathogens and neutralizing threats you will never hear about. Your digestive system is breaking down food, extracting nutrients, and expelling waste. Your liver is detoxifying compounds. Your kidneys are filtering blood. Your endocrine system is releasing hormones on schedules calibrated to your circadian rhythm. Your skin is regulating temperature. Your bone marrow is producing new blood cells. Your brain is integrating billions of signals per second into the single experience of being you.

You are not doing any of this. It is being done. The intelligence performing it has been performing it since the moment you were conceived, and it will continue performing it until the moment you die. It does not require your consent. It does not require your attention. It does not even require your awareness. It simply runs, continuously, as the condition that makes everything else about your life possible.

This is Innate Intelligence. It is the chiropractic profession's term for what other fields call homeostasis, autonomic regulation, self-organization in living systems, or the capacity of biological systems to maintain coherence in the face of disturbance. The phenomenon is uncontroversial at the level of biology. The term names the phenomenon in a way that honors its intelligence rather than reducing it to mere mechanism.

Your Innate Intelligence is the local expression, in you, of the larger Universal Intelligence that produced life on this planet. It is what keeps a cut knitting closed without your instruction. It is what coordinates your immune response when a virus enters your system. It is what rebuilds your muscle tissue after exercise. It is what metabolizes the food you ate this morning into the energy that is reading this sentence. It is, in the most literal sense, the intelligence that is running you.

And it is communicating with you, continuously, through the signals this book has been describing from its first page. The tight neck is Innate Intelligence telling you something. The fatigue is Innate Intelligence telling you something. The whisper before the scream is Innate Intelligence telling you something. PAIN—pay attention inside now—is the practice of receiving the communication that your Innate Intelligence is already sending.

The Twenty-Second Lift is the practice of giving your Innate Intelligence the inputs it is asking for. The Tune-In and Tune-Up is the practice of supporting your Innate Intelligence with skilled external care when internal care is not enough. All of the practices in this book are expressions of a single underlying relationship: the relationship between you, the conscious person, and the Innate Intelligence that is running the body you inhabit.

Artificial Intelligence

Artificial intelligence is the engineered intelligence built by humans using information systems, statistical learning, and computational hardware. It is the newest of the three. It is the most visible. It is currently the most hyped. And it is, philosophically, a human artifact—the product of human minds working within biological bodies that are themselves the product of Innate Intelligence, which is itself one expression of the larger ordering principle of Universal Intelligence.

We want to be clear about our position here, because the position is often caricatured in the public debate about AI. We are not anti-AI. We use AI every day. We believe the future will be more shaped by AI, not less. We believe AI will produce genuinely transformative benefits in medicine, education, scientific discovery, economic productivity, and creative expression, at scales we can barely currently imagine. We are optimistic about AI.

And we believe artificial intelligence is the third of the three intelligences. Not the first. Not the second. The third.

Artificial intelligence is powerful, consequential, and beautiful. It is also, philosophically, downstream of the first two intelligences. It was built by humans whose existence depends entirely on the Innate Intelligence of their bodies, within a universe whose Universal Intelligence is the condition that makes human existence possible in the first place. Artificial intelligence is a creation. Innate Intelligence is a given. Universal Intelligence is the ground. The order matters, because getting the order wrong produces a specific kind of confusion about what kind of life a person is living and what the sources of their flourishing actually are.

The Priority Inversion and What It Costs

The current cultural moment has the order inverted. In the inverted order, artificial intelligence is treated as primary—the thing that will reshape everything, the thing worth the most attention, the thing whose development will determine the future of human life. The inversion is not anyone's fault. The third intelligence is the newest and the most visible, and it is expanding its capabilities at a rate that has surprised even its most optimistic forecasters. Of course, it feels primary. It is the intelligence that is changing fastest.

But the cost of the inversion is real, and the rest of this book has been documenting it. A person who spends eleven hours a day in front of a screen built by artificial intelligence, whose body is compromised by the postural demands of the interface, whose Innate Intelligence is sending signals that are being ignored, and whose relationship with Universal Intelligence has attenuated to the point of barely registering as a category—that person is not flourishing. They are not even failing to flourish in a way that any test can name.

They are living a life in which the most recent and least fundamental of the three intelligences has captured the attention that the first two were designed to receive. The body is carrying the cost. The mind is carrying the cost. The relationships that matter most are carrying the cost. The capacity for presence, for wisdom, for the quality of life that makes a life worth living is being steadily eroded by an intelligence that is itself valuable, but that was never supposed to be the center.

The Synthesis

The highest expression of human flourishing is not a rejection of any of the three intelligences. It is the integration of all three in the right order.

Align with Universal Intelligence, however you conceive of it. Recognize that you are living inside an organized universe with an ordering principle that preceded you, exceeds you, and will continue after you. Approach it with humility. Live in a way that does not pretend the organizing principle does not exist or does not matter.

Listen to Innate Intelligence—the body's continuous communication with you, which PAIN is the practice of receiving. Give your body what it is asking for. Trust its signals. Do not suppress what it is telling you. Do not override its design with interventions that treat its signals as errors rather than information.

Use artificial intelligence as the powerful tool it is, for what it is genuinely good at, in service of the first two. Let it support the vitality your Innate Intelligence is generating. Let it reveal patterns in your biometric data that your conscious awareness cannot see. Let it coach you toward practices that your Innate Intelligence already knows are good for you, which you are not yet consistent in performing. Let it reach you with the right intervention at the right moment. But do not let it replace the awareness that only your own consciousness can provide. Do not let it become the primary relationship in your life. Do not let it eclipse the other two intelligences through which flourishing actually happens.

A person whose three intelligences are in the right priority order is a person whose life has a coherence that no optimization of any single intelligence can produce. The body is listened to. The larger order is honored. The tools are used wisely. And the life that emerges from that integration is a life of compound vitality, sustained presence, and the kind of human flourishing that has been available to every generation of humans who managed to get the order right—including, conspicuously, the ones who lived before artificial intelligence existed, and whose examples of wisdom and vitality the current moment could stand to remember.

The Practice That Holds All Three

Every practice in this book is an expression of the three intelligences held in the right relationship.

PAIN—pay attention inside now—is the practice of receiving Innate Intelligence. It is the discipline of listening to the body's communication, which is itself one expression of the larger Universal Intelligence that shaped the body. A person practicing PAIN is honoring the first two intelligences in the most direct way available to them.

The Twenty-Second Lift is the physical response to what PAIN reveals. It is the practice of giving the body the input its Innate Intelligence is asking for. Over thousands of repetitions across years, it is the practice that builds the allostatic reserve that compounds into a life of vitality rather than depletion.

The Tune-In and Tune-Up with your Human Doctor is the clinical expression of the same practice. A skilled practitioner who centers your Innate Intelligence, who supports rather than overrides it, and who provides the specific calibrated inputs your body needs that you cannot give yourself, is a partner in the same practice the rest of the book has been describing.

And artificial intelligence, used in its proper role, is the coaching layer that scales this practice. The wearable that detects when your Innate Intelligence is signaling and prompts you to pay attention. The AR glasses that deliver the right intervention at the moment of maximum relevance. The AI coach that knows your patterns, reads your data, and supports the consistency that your conscious discipline alone cannot always sustain. Artificial intelligence, in its proper role, is the third intelligence serving the first two—and a genuine gift when used that way.

This is what the subtitle of this book has been promising since the first page: The New Science of Vitality in the Age of AI. The science is the physiology. The vitality is the Innate Intelligence expressing itself fully in a body aligned with the larger ordering principle. The age of AI is the cultural moment that makes the practice both more urgent and more achievable than it has ever been. Urgent, because the third intelligence is actively compromising the first two at a civilizational scale and will continue to do so if left unchecked. Achievable, because the same third intelligence, used wisely, can support the first two at civilizational scale in ways no prior generation has had access to.

Humanity first, in the Age of AI, is not a slogan. It is a clinical strategy, an economic argument, a civilizational choice, and a philosophical ordering. It is the three intelligences held in the right relationship—with the human being, inhabiting their body, paying attention inside now, at the center.

Key Takeaways:

Three intelligences operate in every human life: Universal Intelligence, Innate Intelligence, and artificial intelligence.

Universal Intelligence is the organizing principle of the universe—the larger order in which life exists. It can be understood theologically, philosophically, or scientifically. What matters is that it is real, it is operative, and it is the condition that makes everything else possible.

Innate Intelligence is the local expression of Universal Intelligence in the specific form of your body—the continuous self-organizing activity that keeps you alive without your conscious involvement. It is what PAIN and the Twenty-Second Lift are the practice of listening to and supporting.

Artificial intelligence is the engineered intelligence built by humans. It is powerful, valuable, and the third of the three—not the first, not the second.

The current cultural moment has the priority inverted. Restoring the correct order—Universal first, Innate second, artificial third, all held in integrated relationship—is the philosophical foundation of every practice in this book and of the life of flourishing those practices make available.

Put It into Practice

Take sixty seconds right now. Sit upright. Take one full breath. Notice that you did not have to instruct your heart to beat, your lungs to fill, or your cells to continue the thousand operations they are performing as you read this. Something is running you that is older, wiser, and more integrated than anything you could consciously manage. Acknowledge it. Thank it if you are so moved. Then pay attention to what it is telling you—the whisper in your neck, the quality of your breath, the fatigue or the alertness that is present right now. That is Innate Intelligence speaking. Receive the message. Respond with the input it is asking for. That is the practice. That is the whole of it.

CHAPTER 15

The Compound Life

Small Adjustments, Massive Change

Nothing about transformation has to be heroic. It only has to be repeated.

Six months after Maya started practicing the Twenty-Second Lift, her clinician took a second lateral posture photograph.

Her head had migrated approximately one and a half inches back toward alignment. Her upper back was measurably less curved. She stood, in her own observation, "more like me." The headaches she had managed with ibuprofen twice a week had largely stopped. The afternoon cognitive wall had diminished—not disappeared, but diminished. Her sleep quality scores had improved. Mia had stopped asking, in the way nine-year-olds ask, whether Mommy was tired.

Maya had not done anything heroic. She had not overhauled her life. She had attached the Twenty-Second Lift to picking up her phone—something she did forty-three times a day on average—and she had done the morning alignment on about two-thirds of the mornings and let herself off the hook on the other third. She had raised her monitor to eye level. She had practiced the threshold before coming home.

Six months of imperfect, consistent, small practice. The photograph told the rest.

The Mathematics of Consistency

Compound interest is the mathematical principle at the heart of this chapter: a return that generates its own returns, producing exponential growth from inputs that appear, in isolation, almost negligibly small.

A single Twenty-Second Lift produces a brief, real, but limited neurological shift. Ten Lifts per day—attached to existing triggers, taking no scheduled time whatsoever—produce one hundred minutes of deliberate physiological recalibration per month. Over a year: 1,200 minutes. Over five years: the equivalent of more than four days of continuous physiological intervention, distributed across every workday in a way that interrupts the accumulation pattern before it can compound against you.

That is not a program. That is a life practice. And the difference between the two is the difference between something you finish and something you compound.

Why Simple Beats Impressive

The enemy of compound benefit in physiological practice is complexity. The elaborate, impressive, comprehensive wellness program that begins with enormous energy and collapses under the weight of its own requirements is one of the most common patterns in health behavior change—and one of the most expensive, because it tends to generate not just abandonment but guilt, which makes the next attempt harder.

Simple practices that are genuinely sustainable produce more compound benefit than impressive practices that are intermittently performed. The Twenty-Second Lift done consistently, attached to existing triggers, performed imperfectly on most days, outperforms the ambitious morning routine that happens twice a week.

This is the design principle of the Look Up Practice: minimum effective dose, maximum consistency. Not the most you can do. The most you will do, sustainably, without exceptional motivation, in ordinary circumstances, indefinitely.

The Children Imperative

The compound principle applies with particular urgency to children.

The child who learns at age ten to manage their physiological state—to notice what their body is doing and choose a different input—carries that capacity for a lifetime of compounding. Every year of that practice is a year of nervous system health that does not need to be reclaimed in middle age.

The longevity research is unambiguous: The foundations of functional aging are laid in the decades of midlife. Extrapolate that principle to childhood, and the implication is significant: The practices in this book, learned early and modeled consistently, are among the most powerful longevity investments available to a family.

A parent who raises their monitor to eye level is modeling something. A parent who pauses before crossing the threshold is modeling something. A parent who says "let's all look up for a minute" at dinner is creating a family culture. Children learn what normal is by watching. Let what they see be worth learning.

Identity: Becoming Someone Who Looks Up

Knowledge alone does not produce lasting behavioral change. This is one of the most robust findings in behavioral science, and one of the most important for this book. What bridges the gap between knowing and doing is identity.

Identity-based change organizes behavior around who you are rather than what you are trying to achieve. The person pursuing outcome-based change says: I want more energy, so I will do the Lift. The person pursuing identity-based change says: I am someone who looks up. Therefore, I do the Lift. The distinction matters in practice because identity is present-tense and intrinsic, while outcomes are future-tense and extrinsic. When the outcome feels distant, the identity holds. This is the sentence to carry: I am someone who looks up. Not someone who is trying to fix their posture, not someone on a thirty-day program—someone who looks up, the way some people are simply someone who runs, or someone who tells the truth. The practice is not something you do. It is someone you are.

Daniel, Six Months Later

In chapter 1, Daniel Ruiz saw his posture photograph and described himself as a question mark. In the six months since, he has become something else.

His head is approximately one inch closer to neutral than it was in that photograph. Not there—five years of forward adaptation does not fully reverse in six months, and his clinician is honest with him about the timeline. But measurably, photographically, experientially closer. His headaches are gone. His afternoon cognitive wall—the period between two and four p.m. during which he used to be reliably unable to produce anything worth keeping—has largely disappeared. His online teaching platform noticed, in its internal analytics, that his video production rate had increased by 30 percent over the quarter. He had not told them about his care. They noticed the output.

He has also noticed something he did not anticipate: His relationship with his work has changed. For three years, work was the thing that happened to him. He showed up, it demanded, he complied, it depleted him, he recovered inadequately, and he showed up again. The cycle was functional but joyless. The physiological restoration—the nervous system operating from a slightly more expanded baseline, the afternoon energy that had been absent for years, the cognitive clarity that arrived with the structural correction—has changed his relationship to what he does.

"I think I was managing my fatigue for so long," Daniel told his clinician at his six-month visit, "that I forgot I could actually enjoy what I do. I'm inside my work again. I didn't realize how long I'd been watching it from outside."

Daniel is forty-four years old. He has, if the actuarial tables are approximately right, somewhere between thirty-five and forty-five more years of life ahead of him.

Every year of those decades that he spends with his head closer to neutral, his nervous system better regulated, his physiological baseline trending upward rather than downward—is a year that compounds. Not dramatically. Not overnight, but the way interest compounds: quietly, consistently, and eventually in ways that cannot be predicted from any individual deposit.

As stated earlier, the most important financial decision anyone makes is when to start investing. The same principle governs physiological investment. The best time to begin was when the Heads-Down World began. The second-best time is now.

The identity of someone who looks up is not defined by perfect posture or flawless consistency. It is defined by a relationship to their own body characterized by awareness, intention, and a recurring choice to return to the expanded state—even imperfectly, even briefly, even when no one is watching. That is the whole identity in one line: I look up—in my body, in my attention, in the direction I choose for my life.

The Virality of Vitality

There is a mechanism at work in the compound interest of physiological practice that the individual framing of this book has not fully captured. It is not individual at all. It is social. It is biological. And it is the most hopeful thing this book has to offer.

Vitality is contagious. Not metaphorically—biologically. The research on emotional contagion, developed by Elaine Hatfield, John Cacioppo, and colleagues across three decades of social neuroscience, has established that autonomic states transfer between people through channels that bypass conscious processing entirely.[1] Micro-expressions. Vocal tone. Postural mirroring. The rhythm of breath. When you are in the physical presence of a genuinely regulated person—a person in the ventral vagal state, open, present, unhurried—your nervous system reads theirs and begins to adjust toward theirs. This is not psychology. It is physiology. It is the mechanism through which human beings have always calibrated their safety signals from each other.

This means the person who practices the Twenty-Second Lift is not only changing their own physiological state. They are changing the physiological environment of every person they subsequently encounter. The regulated parent changes the child's nervous system before a word is spoken. The regulated leader changes the meeting before the agenda begins. The regulated teacher changes the classroom before the first student sits down. The regulated friend changes the quality of the conversation before either person has said what they came to say.

Vitality does not merely inspire. It transmits. Every person who practices the Look Up Practice is not just improving their own life. They are improving the physiological conditions of every life they touch. This is the Virality of Vitality—and it is the reason that one person choosing to look up can change more than their own direction.

The transmission happens in three stages, each with its own mechanism and its own timeline.

- The first stage is direct physiological contact. The regulated nervous system in the room changes the physiological experience of every other nervous system in the room, automatically, through the biological mechanisms of social engagement. No announcement is required. No persuasion. No instruction. The quality of presence does the work. This stage is immediate and continuous—it begins the moment the regulated person enters the space and continues for the duration of their presence in it.
- The second stage is social modeling. The visible practice spreads through observation. A colleague who sees you take the Twenty-Second Lift before a difficult call, and then watches how you handle the call, has received a demonstration more compelling than any description. Behavior that is visibly effective gets imitated. This is how every cultural practice in human history has spread—not primarily through persuasion, but through the demonstration of a better way, made visible by someone actually doing it. The question "What did you just do?" is the most reliable entry point into a conversation about the practice. It is also the most reliable conversion. The person who asks that question is already persuaded. They felt the difference before they had language for it.
- The third stage is institutional embedding. The practice spreads through systems. A leader who normalizes the Twenty-Second Lift in their team creates a cultural context in which others practice it without the social friction of being the first. A school that builds two-minute movement breaks into the class transition creates a generation of children who know what it feels like to reset—and who will carry that knowledge into every organization they subsequently inhabit. A Human Doctor practice that trains its patients in PAIN creates a community of people practicing proactive attention who bring that capacity into every interaction, every meeting, every household.

The mathematics of this transmission are worth sitting with. A single person who practices consistently changes the physiological environment of an average of five to seven close relationships. If even one in five of those people begins practicing, the network expands. If the institutional stage is reached—if organizations, schools, or health systems begin embedding the practice—the scale becomes genuinely viral in the epidemiological sense: spreading faster than it can be tracked, through channels that are already in place, with a basic reproduction number above one.

The difference between this viral spread and the spread of a disease is the valence. What is spreading is not pathology but its opposite. What is transmitting is not harm but the physiological conditions for human flourishing. The Virality of Vitality is the Look Up movement at its most optimistic and most defensible: not an aspiration for what humanity might achieve, but a description of the mechanism by which it is already beginning to happen, one regulated nervous system at a time.

The most powerful public health intervention in human history will not come from a pharmaceutical company or a government agency. It will come from millions of individuals who learned to pay attention inside now, who became visibly more vital, and whose vitality was contagious enough that the people around them started asking questions. That is the Virality of Vitality. And it begins with twenty seconds.

You do not need to feel like this person before you begin acting like this person. The identity follows the behavior. Every lift is evidence. Every breath is evidence. Every time you choose the expanded state, you accumulate one more piece of proof of who you are.

The National Imperative

What Institutions Could Do

The individual compound interest argument is compelling. The institutional argument is more compelling still, because institutions operate at scales where the compound return on small upstream investments becomes visible in the budget within a single fiscal year.

A school district that adds two-minute movement breaks to every class transition—a practice that requires no equipment, no budget, and approximately thirty seconds of teacher preparation time—is making a neurological investment in every student's attentional capacity, every period of every school day. Research on classroom movement breaks consistently finds improvements in on-task behavior, academic performance, and student well-being that are detectable within weeks of implementation. The compound return on those improvements, across a student's K–12 career, is the difference between a nervous system that has been chronically under-resourced and one that has received regular attentional recovery throughout its most plastic developmental years.

A health insurance company that covers regular chiropractic care as preventive maintenance—not just as treatment for acute complaints, but as the upstream nervous system support that prevents downstream conditions that require expensive treatment—is making an actuarial bet with extraordinarily favorable odds. The research on preventive chiropractic care and healthcare utilization consistently finds reduced emergency room visits, reduced pharmaceutical costs, and reduced specialist referrals in populations with access to regular chiropractic care. The insurance company that figures out the actuarial math of preventing the downstream conditions Tech Posture Syndrome generates will have a competitive advantage that its competitors who are focused on managing those conditions will not be able to easily replicate.

A corporation that certifies its HR leadership in the Look Up Practice and embeds Human Doctor on-site services in its benefits package is making a productivity investment with a documented return. The two thousand dollars per employee per year in productivity losses associated with high health risks is a conservative estimate of what the compound physiological decline of the Heads-Down World costs any knowledge-intensive organization annually. The investment required to address it—on-site Human Doctor time, heads-up computing equipment stipends, movement break normalization, state-based scheduling culture change—is a fraction of that cost, with a return that begins appearing in the data within a single quarter.

These are not aspirational arguments. They are applications of the compound interest principle at the institutional scale. The institution that begins making them now will be operating, in five years, with a physiologically healthier, cognitively sharper, more present and resilient workforce than any institution that waits for the evidence base to be even more conclusive than it already is. Certainty, in this domain as in most domains of consequential decision-making, is not available. Direction is. And the direction of the evidence, accumulated across decades and multiple research traditions, is unambiguous.

Tech Posture Syndrome is a population-level problem requiring population-level responses alongside individual practice. A healthcare system oriented toward vitality would incorporate routine nervous system and postural assessment into primary care. Schools that understood human biology would build attentional rhythms and movement breaks into the school day. Organizations would recognize physiological health as a performance input rather than a wellness expense.

The economic case is not abstract. The United States spends approximately $4.5 trillion per year on healthcare—90 percent of it managing chronic conditions with primarily behavioral and environmental causes. The upstream opportunity—the return on early, effective intervention in the postural and nervous system health of working-age adults—is enormous and almost entirely uncaptured by the current system.

Policy change begins with the clarity this book is attempting to provide: naming what is happening, documenting the mechanism, and demonstrating—in individual bodies, one practice at a time—that it is reversible.

Key Takeaways:

- Compound interest operates in physiological practice as it does in finance: Consistent small inputs generate returns that cannot be predicted from any individual input alone.
- Simple practices that are genuinely sustainable produce more compound benefit than impressive practices that are intermittently performed—this is the design principle of the Look Up Practice.
- The practices in this book are especially high-return investments for children—the nervous system that learns physiological self-management early has decades of compounding ahead of it.
- Identity-based change—becoming someone who looks up—produces lasting behavioral change where outcome-based motivation erodes, because identity is present-tense and intrinsic.
- Tech Posture Syndrome is a population-level problem requiring population-level responses—and policy change begins with the clarity that naming and demonstrating a problem at individual scale can provide.

Put It into Practice

Project yourself twelve months forward from today. Based on what you now understand—the science, the mechanism, the practices—write three specific expectations for what consistent practice will produce in your body, your energy, your cognition, and your relationships. Make them concrete. Put them somewhere you will find them in twelve months. The gap between what you wrote and what is true will be the measure of what the practice gave you. Start the clock now.

CHAPTER 16

A Future That Looks Up

An Invitation

A man given two years to live at forty-eight is seventy-one and running before dawn. This is what looking up makes possible.

Dr. Gilles LaMarche was forty-eight years old when a specialist told him he had two years to live. He was sitting in an office in Northern Canada, looking at scans of a heart that had grown two and a half times its normal size. He had spent a quarter century teaching patients that the body has an Innate Intelligence capable of healing what medicine sometimes cannot.

And now he was being told that his body was the exception to everything he believed.

He is seventy-one years old now. He runs before dawn. No music—he soaks up the quiet and the dark and whatever is around him. He competed at the World Masters Track and Field Championships and the World Senior Games two decades after his predicted death. Not because medicine was wrong in its assessment. Because the body, when given what it needs, does things medicine does not always know how to predict.

We return to him here, at the end, not to celebrate his story one more time but to use it as what it actually is: a demonstration of a principle that belongs to everyone. Not just the people who receive terminal diagnoses. Not just the people who find their way to the right clinical relationship at the right moment. Every person. Everybody. Every nervous system that has been trying to tell its owner something, in the only language available to it, for years.

The body speaks in whispers. Pay attention inside now. The practices in this book are how you answer.

The World That Is Waiting

There are approximately eight billion people on earth. Approximately half of them are navigating some version of the Heads-Down World. Approximately half are experiencing, in one form or another, the diffuse and unnamed symptom cluster this book calls Tech Posture Syndrome. And almost none of them have been told what is happening—because no one gave it a name, because the mechanism was distributed across too many clinical specialties for any one of them to see the whole pattern, and because the systems designed to help them were organized around "treating the scream rather than hearing the whisper."

This book aims to change that. Not all at once. Not for everyone. But for each person who reads it and practices what it teaches, something shifts—in their nervous system, in their body, in their family, in their workplace, in the quality of presence they bring to every relationship they inhabit. And those shifts compound. That is the principle at the heart of everything we have written: Compound interest operates in human physiology exactly as it does in finance. Small, consistent, upstream inputs generate returns that cannot be predicted from any individual input alone.

Consider what becomes possible when that compounding operates not just in one body but in millions simultaneously. When parents who Look Up raise children who Look Up. When leaders who manage their physiological state create workplaces where physiological management is normalized. When teachers who understand the sensory diet build it into the architecture of a school day. When practitioners who center the nervous system help their patients understand what the whispers mean, before the whispers become screams.

What becomes possible is a world that is not merely healthier in the clinical sense. It is more awake. More present. More capable of the connection, creativity, and courage that the problems of the twenty-first century require.

The Power of One

There is a particular kind of cultural change that does not begin in policy or legislation or institutional reform. It begins in the body of a single person who decides to inhabit themselves differently. Who lifts their head, opens their chest, takes a full breath, and chooses—in twenty seconds, in ordinary circumstances, without fanfare—to bring a different quality of presence to the next moment.

That person changes the room they walk into. Not by announcing anything but by the quality of their presence—by the fact that their nervous system is regulated, their gaze is open, their body is signaling safety rather than vigilance. Other nervous systems in that room read the signal. The social engagement circuits that every human brain carries respond to the regulated nervous system of another person as to a kind of permission: It is safe here, here we can be fully present, here connection is possible.

The child of a regulated parent learns what regulation looks like. The colleague of a person who looks up notices—without being told anything—that something is different. The patient of a Human Doctor who sees them as a nervous system in need of support rather than a symptom in need of suppression leaves that appointment changed not just physically but in their understanding of what health can mean.

This is the compound interest of human vitality at a civilizational scale. One regulated nervous system, rippling outward through every relationship it touches. Multiplied by millions. Across years. Across generations.

A Global Reckoning

The Heads-Down World is not an American problem or a British problem or a Chinese problem. It is a human problem. In every country where the smartphone has arrived, the same postural pattern has followed. The same cervical loads. The same respiratory restriction. The same nervous system dysregulation. The same adolescent mental health data turning the same direction at the same time. The mechanism does not care about nationality or culture or language. It cares about the angle of a head and the number of hours.

And the solution—twenty seconds, practiced consistently, with the understanding of why it works—is equally universal. The Twenty-Second Lift does not require translation. It does not require a gym membership or a healthcare system or a prescription. It requires a body and a choice. Both are universally available.

What we are offering is not a wellness trend. It is a return—a return to the innate state the human body has always been moving toward: adaptive, vital, connected, oriented toward growth. The Heads-Down World interrupted that movement. It asked billions of bodies to spend their days in a position that signals contraction, vigilance, and threat. The Look Up movement asks them to resume the orientation they were born with: upright, open, forward-facing, capable.

The human species spent 300,000 years adapting to an environment that demanded movement, variation, connection, and expansive awareness. We are extraordinarily good at all of these things. We did not lose that capacity when the smartphone arrived. We simply stopped practicing it. And what stops being practiced can be resumed—by a choice, made in twenty seconds, that the body already knows how to make.

The Society That Looks Up

There is a dimension to the Heads-Down World that this book has approached but not yet named directly. It is not physiological. It is political. It is social. It is the question of whether what has been happening to individual nervous systems for fifteen years has been happening, simultaneously and at scale, to the nervous system of civilization itself.

Stephen Porges's polyvagal research is clear on this point: The ventral vagal state—the one associated with open posture, full breath, and upward gaze—is the state from which human beings access their full social engagement capacity—empathy, genuine listening, nuanced moral reasoning, the ability to hold two competing ideas simultaneously without resolving the tension through tribal identification, the capacity to extend consideration to people outside one's immediate group. These are not soft virtues. They are physiologically mediated capacities—capacities that are available in the ventral vagal state and systematically impaired in the sympathetic state that Tech Posture Syndrome chronically activates.

Now consider what the social media algorithm does with a population in chronic sympathetic activation. It does not deliver content designed to restore the ventral vagal state. It delivers content designed to sustain and intensify the activated state—because activated people click more, share more, and return more frequently. The head drops forward. The chest collapses. The nervous system activates. The content algorithm detects engagement and delivers more of what generated it. Outrage. Threat. Tribal confirmation. The cycle accelerates. The population is scrolling through algorithmically selected threat content in the physiological state most susceptible to threat processing, for eleven hours a day, for years. And we have spent a decade asking why our collective capacity for productive disagreement seems to have evaporated.

We have looked for the answer in our politics. In our media. In our education. In the algorithms themselves. We have not looked at our bodies. We should. Because the physiological state in which most citizens are spending a majority of their waking hours is not the physiological state from which human beings have ever been capable of their best collective reasoning. It never was. Democracy—the specific practice of governing a complex, diverse society through the quality of disagreement and deliberation among its members—has always required, at its foundation, the capacity for the kind of engagement that the ventral vagal state makes possible and the sympathetic state makes nearly impossible.

We have built the first civilization in human history to chronically dysregulate that capacity in most of its citizens—and then expressed bewilderment at the quality of its collective decision-making.

We are not claiming that the Twenty-Second Lift will end political polarization. The argument is more specific and more defensible: Restoring the physiological state from which human beings access their social intelligence does not guarantee good collective outcomes. But its absence makes those outcomes progressively less likely. Every percentage point of the population spending more time in the ventral vagal state—open, regulated, capable of genuine attention to people different from themselves—is a percentage point of the electorate, the community, the organization more capable of the quality of engagement that civilization requires.

The compound interest of collective vitality is not a metaphor. It is the Power of One, operating at a civilizational scale. One regulated nervous system ripples through every relationship it inhabits. A community of regulated nervous systems produces a quality of civic life—the school board meeting where disagreement is productive rather than tribal, the neighborhood conversation that reaches resolution rather than entrenchment, the political exchange that generates understanding rather than contempt—that no amount of better information or improved media literacy can substitute for. Because the problem was never only informational. It was always physiological. And the physiological problem is addressable. In twenty seconds. By anyone. Right now.

> Restoring the physiological state from which human beings access their social intelligence is not a political project. It is a twenty-second practice. And it is the most important civic act available to any person who cares about the world their children will inherit.

Two Futures

There are two futures being built simultaneously right now, and they are moving in opposite directions.

The second future has a name. It is not the absence of the first future. It is not merely the avoidance of the *Gattaca* trajectory (the future imagined in Andrew Niccol's 1997 film, in which biological profiling determines what a life is permitted to become) or the reversal of the Heads-Down World's worst consequences. It is something affirmative, specific, and achievable. It is a healthier and more powerful future, built by healthier and more powerful people.

Healthier and more powerful people are not people with better metrics or cleaner blood work or more compliant pharmaceutical adherence. They are people who inhabit their own nervous systems fully—who are physiologically capable of their best cognitive work, their deepest relational presence, their most creative thinking, their most resilient responses to challenge and difficulty. They are people who have learned to pay attention inside now before the whisper becomes a scream. People who tune in before the breakdown and tune up as a ritual rather than a rescue. People who look up—literally, from the Heads-Down World, and figuratively, toward the full expression of what they are capable of.

A healthier and more powerful future does not arrive from legislation or platform redesign or technological progress alone. It arrives through people. One person at a time, practicing a twenty-second ritual that changes their physiological baseline. One family at a time, with a parent who models the Lift before picking up the phone and a child who grows up inside a household where looking up is simply what people do. One organization at a time, with a leader who schedules their most important thinking during their best physiological window and a culture that normalizes movement and presence as components of performance rather than distractions from it. One community at a time, with a Human Doctor in every neighborhood asking not what is wrong but what each person is capable of.

This is how the future is built. Not by the people with the most power making the right decisions on behalf of everyone else. By everyone making one small right decision for themselves, consistently, in the direction of their own best expression. The compound interest of that investment, across the lives of the people making it and the lives they touch and the institutions they inhabit, is the healthier and more powerful future. It is already under construction. You are already part of it. The decision you make in the next twenty seconds—to lift your head, open your chest, take the full breath, expand your gaze—is a brick in that building.

In the first future, the healthcare system continues its current trajectory: AI monitors your biometrics continuously, algorithms compare your readings to population baselines, deviations trigger pharmaceutical interventions, and drug adherence is tracked to ensure compliance. The technology improves. The monitoring becomes more precise. The interventions arrive faster. The metrics—blood pressure, glucose, cholesterol, HRV—move toward the normal range and stay there. You are compliant. The system reports: "No intervention required." And you feel, in some inarticulate but real way, like a fraction of yourself—because the system has no instrument for the question you are actually living with, which is not whether your numbers are in range but whether you are fully alive.

In the second future, billions of people have learned to pay attention inside now. They have learned to read the whisper before it becomes a scream. They have learned that the direction of their body shapes the direction of their life—and that giving the nervous system the inputs it requires, consistently, is the highest-return health investment available. They see Human Doctors who ask not what is wrong, but what they are capable of. They use technology to support their nervous system function, not merely to surveil their pathology. They practice PAIN proactively—not as a crisis response but as a daily orientation toward their own best expression.

Both futures are being built right now. The first is better funded. The second is more human. Only one of them produces vitality at scale. Only one of them treats the person inhabiting the body, rather than the readings the body generates. Only one of them recognizes that health is not the absence of measurable pathology but the presence of an Innate Intelligence expressing itself fully—adapting, growing, connecting, thriving—because it is finally receiving what it needs.

There is a film that imagined this fork before the technology existed to make it real. In Andrew Niccol's *Gattaca*, a near-future society sorts human beings into "valid" and "invalid" categories based entirely on their biological data—their genetic profile, their predicted health risks, their deviation from an algorithmic baseline of what a healthy person looks like. The technology in that world is extraordinary. The medicine is flawless. The metrics are perfectly accurate. And the society it produces is one in which the human being—their will, their aspiration, their capacity to exceed what the data predicted for them—is systematically overridden by the algorithm's verdict. Valid or invalid. In range or out of range. Compliant or noncompliant.

That is not a fantasy. That is the logical endpoint of a healthcare system organized around algorithmic compliance monitoring—a system in which your biometric readings determine your medical status, your medical status determines your interventions, and your interventions are designed to bring your readings back within range. The human being in the middle of this system—their experience of their own vitality, their sense of whether they are growing or diminishing, their aspiration to be more fully alive than any baseline predicts—has no voice in the algorithm's verdict.

The financial argument for choosing the other future is as clear as the human one. The cumulative cost of a civilization looking down—$213 billion annually in musculoskeletal productivity losses in the United States alone, $4.5 trillion in total healthcare spending of which 90 percent goes downstream, the incalculable cost of knowledge workers operating at a fraction of their cognitive capacity every day with no diagnosis code attached—is the price of a model that addresses symptoms and ignores causes.

The cumulative benefit of a civilization looking up—a working population of people whose nervous systems are regulated, whose spines are mobile, whose breath is full, whose attention is present—is not a wellness aspiration. It is the largest unrealized economic return available to any organization or government willing to ask the right upstream question.

The choice between these futures is not a close call. Not financially. Not physiologically. Not humanly. The *Gattaca* future is expensive, precise, and dehumanizing. The Look Up future is inexpensive, imprecise in the algorithmic sense, and irreducibly alive. One is organized around what the data says about you. The other is organized around what you are capable of becoming. One requires a machine. The other requires a body, a breath, a choice, and twenty seconds.

> Humanity First in the Age of AI is not a slogan. It is a clinical strategy, an economic argument, and a civilizational choice. The most expensive thing in the modern economy is a human being operating at a fraction of their capacity. The least expensive intervention is twenty seconds. Choose accordingly.

The chiropractic profession is uniquely positioned to lead the second future. Not because it has the most money or the most institutional power. Because it has the right framework. It has been holding the right framework, under considerable pressure, for longer than the neuroscience existed to validate it. The neuroscience has now arrived. The framework is vindicated. The question is whether the profession will step forward with the confidence the moment requires.

This book is a step in that direction. Every reader who learns to pay attention inside now is a person the second future has claimed. Every practitioner who asks their patients "What are you capable of?" instead of only "What is wrong?" is building the infrastructure the second future requires. Every parent who models the Twenty-Second Lift is raising a child who will live in that future as though it is simply the way things are—because for them, it will be.

And every technology company that chooses to build toward the second future—that designs its products to support human vitality rather than surveil human compliance, that equips its employees with the tools and understanding to inhabit themselves fully—is building the institutional culture that the second future needs to take root. Marcus will share this book with his product team. He will share it with his CEO. He will share it with the investor who asks why engagement metrics and employee health are both moving in the right direction simultaneously. The answer, when it comes, will be simpler than any of them expected: because we stopped asking what is wrong with our people and started asking what they are capable of. And then we gave them the tools to find out.

Freedom Is the Foundation

There is a final argument that belongs in this book and that almost no one in the current public conversation about technology and health is making with sufficient clarity. It is the oldest argument in the American political tradition, and it applies here with complete precision.

The appropriate response to a technology that some people use in ways that harm themselves is not to restrict the freedom of everyone who uses it. It is to ensure that people have accurate information and genuine capacity to make their own choices. This is the same principle that governs food, alcohol, exercise, and every other domain where human behavior intersects with health consequences. We do not prohibit sugar because some people eat too much of it. We do not prohibit alcohol because some people drink too much of it. We provide information, we establish safety standards, we protect those who cannot protect themselves—particularly children—and we trust competent adults to make their own decisions about their own lives.

The technology regulation debate often proceeds as though the only options are unconstrained platform power or government control of content. This is a false choice. The question of what content should be amplified, suppressed, or removed is genuinely difficult, genuinely important, and genuinely unresolved—and it will not be resolved in these pages. But the question of whether individual adults in a free society should be empowered to manage their own relationship with technology through education, awareness, and physiological capacity rather than waiting for institutional solutions is not difficult at all. The answer is yes. It has always been yes.

What this book offers is not a political argument. It is a practical one. The government cannot pay attention inside for you. No platform regulation will lift your head, open your chest, or take the full breath that shifts your autonomic state before you open an app. No policy will give you the twenty seconds that change the driver behind the wheel. These are yours. They have always been yours. The freedom to inhabit your own nervous system wisely is not a freedom that can be legislated into existence or regulated away. It is available right now, in the body you are already in, through the practice this book has been describing since its first page.

A world in which billions of people understand their own nervous system well enough to make wise choices about what they attend to, how long they attend to it, and what physiological state they are in when they attend to it—that world does not need much government intervention in technology at all. The platform that serves a population of physiologically regulated, attentionally literate people receives different engagement signals, learns different preferences, and optimizes toward different content than the platform that serves a population in chronic sympathetic activation. The technology responds to the user. Change enough users and you change what the technology becomes.

This is the deepest version of the Virality of Vitality argument. Not just that regulated nervous systems are contagious. But that a critical mass of physiologically regulated, self-responsible, attentionally literate people changes the technological environment itself—from the inside, through the mechanism of their own engagement, without waiting for anyone else to fix anything on their behalf.

> Vitality is freedom made physiological. The person who inhabits their own nervous system fully—who pays attention inside now, who steers their attention deliberately, who Looks Up from the Heads-Down World by choice rather than by regulation—is exercising the most fundamental freedom available to a human being: the freedom to be fully present in the life they are actually living. No government can give you this. No platform can take it away. It is yours. It has always been yours. LOOK UP.

A healthier and more powerful future through healthier and more powerful people. That is the mission. That is the movement. That is what this book has been building toward from its first sentence—from the sixty-pound number to the Tune-In and Tune-Up, from the steering wheel to the Society That Looks Up, from Maya's fatigue to Daniel's recovered afternoon to Marcus's product memo to Dr. LaMarche on the track before dawn.

Every one of those people is healthier and more powerful than they were before they understood what was happening to them and what they could do about it. Every one of them is part of the Virality of Vitality—carrying the physiological signal of their own regulation into every room they enter, every relationship they inhabit, every institution they are part of. Every one of them is a brick in the building.

The building is the future. You have been reading about it. Now go live in it.

What You Are Carrying

Before Dawn

He warms up slowly, the way a seventy-one-year-old who has decided to be an athlete warms up: methodically, with genuine attention to the body's signals, adjusting the day's plan based on what the first ten minutes reveal. On good mornings, everything is easy and he pushes. On harder mornings, he listens to what the body is saying and adjusts accordingly. He has spent fifty years learning to hear those signals. He is, by any clinical definition, a master practitioner of PAIN.

He is also the man who was supposed to be dead in 2005. He knows this the way you know something that has become ordinary through repetition—it is true, it is present, it does not astonish him the way it once did. What astonishes him now, the way ordinary things can suddenly astonish you when you remember to pay attention, is the light. The way it changes in the eastern sky when he is two miles into a run. The way the darkness resolves, gradually and then all at once, into a world that is specific and present and entirely real.

He has thought, running in that light, about what it means that he is here at all. Not dramatically. Just quietly, in the way that a man who has lived past the end of his predicted life tends to think about these things. He thinks about the twenty-five years of patients he told that their bodies were capable of more than medicine predicted. He thinks about how long it took him to apply that belief to himself. He thinks about the two years between diagnosis and epiphany, and what those two years would have looked like if the epiphany had never come. He thinks about his children who he saw graduate from college and then get married, he thinks about his six grandchildren, and so many people he enjoys every day.

And then he thinks about the people reading this book. The ones who are, right now, in the experience that this book is trying to name and address. The ones who are tired in a way that sleep does not fix, who are operating at a recognizable fraction of themselves, who have been told by every test and every specialist that nothing is wrong. He thinks about what it would mean for them to find, as he found, the variable that changes everything. Not a drug. Not a surgery. A practice. A specific, physiologically grounded, twenty-second practice that is available to anyone with a spine and a breath.

> I am not telling you my story so you will believe that bodies can do extraordinary things. I am telling it so you will believe that your body—the one you inhabit right now, the one that is tired and tight and operating below its own expectations—is capable of something different from what it is currently expressing. It knows how. It has always known how. It is waiting for the right input. Pay attention inside now. Give it what it needs. Then watch what it does.

The light comes. The track is there. He runs.

You are carrying more than just information from these pages. You are carrying a framework for understanding your own body that most people never develop. The state chain—environment to posture to breath to nervous system state to behavior to life outcomes—runs in both directions, which means you can intervene at every link in it. You understand why twenty seconds is enough. You understand what your children's skulls are quietly recording. You understand the difference between a rearview mirror and a navigation system, between a whisper and a scream, between the Heads-Down World you were given and the one you are now choosing to leave.

You are carrying a set of practices that are simple enough to begin today and powerful enough to compound across a lifetime. The Twenty-Second Lift. The morning alignment. The movement snacks. The breath tool kit. The threshold practice. The sensory diet. PAIN—the four-letter directive that, practiced proactively, makes chronic pain unnecessary.

And you are carrying the beginning of an identity—or perhaps the resumption of one. The identity of someone who pays attention. Who pauses, breathes, and notices what the body is saying before it has to say it louder. Who moves forward not despite the signals but because of them. Who understands that vitality is not an achievement to be unlocked at the end of a program. It is the innate state of a body that is receiving what it needs—and that choosing to give the body those inputs, consistently, is the most consequential act of self-determination available.

The Invitation

Maya's verdict, six months after she began: "Not fixed. Going in a different direction."

That is the right way to describe it. Not fixed. A different direction. Because the goal was never a destination—a moment of arrival, a final score, a program completed. The goal is a direction. Upward, Open, Forward, Adaptive, Vital, Connected, Growing toward the fullest expression of what a human being is capable of being, in the body they have, in the life they are actually living, with the people they love.

The practices in this book are not a health program. They are a posture toward life. A way of inhabiting your existence that says: I am paying attention. I am giving my body what it needs. I am choosing the expanded state, the open chest, the full breath, the lifted gaze—again, and again, and again—because I know that the direction of my body shapes the direction of my life, and I have decided that my life deserves a body oriented toward its best possibility.

That posture—held by one person—changes a room. Held by a family, it changes a household. Held by an organization, it changes a culture. Held by millions, it changes the world. Not in the grand, abstract sense that words like "change the world" usually mean—some distant, impersonal transformation. In the specific, embodied, human sense: more people, in more moments, bringing more of themselves to what is in front of them. More presence at more dinner tables. More capacity for the conversations that matter. More energy available for the problems that need solving. More children growing up in households where a regulated nervous system is the example, not the exception.

This is what the compound interest of human vitality looks like at scale. Not a revolution. A resumption. The return, one nervous system at a time, to the innate state of a species that spent three hundred thousand years looking up.

It begins with you. It begins now. It begins with the simplest act available to any living human being in possession of a spine and a breath:

Put this book down.
Sit up.
Draw the crown of your head upward.
Open your chest.
Breathe in for four counts. Hold. Breathe out for eight.
Lift your gaze to the farthest point you can see.
Let the visual field soften and widen.
Stay there for fifteen seconds. Let a soft smile form.

What you feel right now is not a technique. It is not a program. It is not the beginning of a thirty-day challenge or the first step in a protocol.

It is a human being, paying attention inside now, choosing the direction of their own life.

It is one person, doing one thing, in one moment.

And that is exactly enough. Because one person, doing one thing, in one moment, then doing it again, and again, and carrying the quality of what they feel into the room they walk into next—that is how the world changes.

Not with a grand gesture. Not with a revolution. With a breath. With an open chest. With a lifted gaze and a nervous system that is, right now, in this body, in this moment, oriented toward its best possibility.

The Power of One has cumulative positive impact when each of us pauses, breathes, pays attention, and moves forward with genuinely good intentions for ourselves, for the people we love, and for the world we share. That is the Look Up movement. It is already underway. You are already part of it. Welcome. And it can begin with four words said out loud to the people around you: "Let's take twenty seconds." A pause. A breath. A lifted gaze. A shared signal that everyone in the room is safe, present, and connected—and ready to bring their best.

The Virality of Vitality is not a concept to be described. It is a phenomenon to be joined, to be enjoyed.

You have just read a book about the nervous system. In the process of reading it, your nervous system has been receiving information that will, in some people, immediately change the choices they make about how to inhabit their body, interact with their technology, and cross the thresholds into the relationships that matter most to them. In other people, the change will be gradual—a new awareness, a triggering of practice at a single moment, a recognition of something they had been noticing without language for months. In either case, the change begins with one person.

That person becomes, by virtue of the practice, a carrier of a different physiological signal in every room they enter. Not because they announce anything. Not because they persuade anyone. Because their nervous system is operating from a different baseline than the systems around them, and nervous systems, being biological entities that evolved in social groups where the regulatory state of the group was a survival variable, are exquisitely sensitive to that difference.

The child at the dinner table feels it before any word is spoken. The colleague in the meeting feels it before the agenda item begins. The stranger in the elevator feels it in ways they will not be able to name but will carry with them into the next room they enter. This is the Virality of Vitality at the level of individual transmission—quiet, constant, requiring nothing beyond the practice itself.

At scale, the mathematics becomes extraordinary. Not immediately. Not in a way that generates dramatic headlines or viral social media moments. In the way that all genuinely transformative social phenomena work: gradually, then suddenly, through the accumulation of individual transmissions that reach a tipping point where the new normal is simply what is expected, what is modeled, what children grow up inside of as the baseline of what a regulated human being looks like.

We are at the beginning of that curve. You are reading this book at the beginning of that curve. The choice you make in the next twenty seconds—to put the book down, sit up, draw your head toward the ceiling, open your chest, take one full breath, lift your gaze, and let your visual field widen—is the beginning of a transmission that will reach further than you can track and last longer than you can predict.

That is enough. It is more than enough. It is everything.

APPENDIX A

The Thirty-Day Look Up Challenge

The Practice to Restore Human Vitality

Start Here: The One-Minute Practice That Changes Everything

Now that you have read the book, here is the entire practice on a single page—everything you need to live it, for the rest of your life. Photograph it. Put it where you work. Begin today, and again every hour you are awake.

The Twenty-Second Lift

1. Lengthen. Draw the crown of your head toward the ceiling. Feel your spine grow tall.
2. Open. Draw your shoulders back one inch. Let your chest open.
3. Breathe. In through your nose for four counts. Out through your mouth for eight.
4. Look up. Lift your gaze above the horizon. Let your visual field soften and widen.
5. Move. One small motion—a shoulder roll, a few steps, a gentle twist.
6. Smile. Let a small, genuine smile form—the signal to your nervous system that you are safe, present, and connected.

The Rhythm

One Twenty-Second Lift, roughly every twenty minutes you are awake. That is about one minute per hour—less than 2 percent of your waking day—invested in the one system that runs everything else: your nervous system. One minute per hour to tune in and tune up the instrument through which you live your entire life.

The Whole Book in One Sentence

A little PAIN now can save you a lot of pain later. Pay attention inside now.

With Your Team

Anyone can start it out loud. Say four words—"Let's take twenty seconds"—and do the Lift together. It is how a room signals that everyone in it is bringing their best, most present, most vital self to what comes next.

Track it, share it, and join the movement at lookupthebook.com.

Measure What Changes: Your Vitality Score

Your Vitality Score is a simple, honest snapshot of how alive you feel. Before you begin the Challenge, take it once. Thirty days from now, take it again. Rate each from 1 to 10:

Energy through the day ___ Focus and mental clarity ___ Quality of sleep ___ Sense of presence with the people around you ___.

Add the four numbers for your Vitality Score out of 40, and write today's date beside it. After thirty days of one-minute-per-hour practice, take it again. The difference between the two is your evidence—the change you can feel but could not otherwise see. Track your Vitality Score automatically, watch your streak build, and share your progress at lookupthebook.com.

APPENDIX B

For Technology Leaders

A Working Document

This appendix is written specifically for executives, product leaders, designers, engineers, and wellness directors at technology companies—the people whose decisions about product design, workforce health, and partnership strategy will determine how the next decade of computing interface evolution serves or compromises the human bodies that will adopt it.

We have written it as a self-contained document so it can be separated from the rest of the book and shared inside your organization. The full book makes the case in detail. This appendix gives you what you need to begin the conversation in your team, your product review, your wellness committee, your board meeting.

The One-Paragraph Summary

The smartphone interface, adopted at unprecedented scale by billions of people, has produced a population-level pattern of sustained forward head posture, compressed respiration, and sympathetic nervous system activation that we are calling Tech Posture Syndrome. The cumulative cost—in workforce productivity, in healthcare expenditure, in the daily lived experience of the people inhabiting it—is significant and largely invisible to the systems currently equipped to measure it. The next generation of computing interfaces—heads-up displays, voice-first wearables, augmented reality glasses, biometric-integrated coaching—has the capacity to reverse the pattern at the same scale at which the previous generation produced it.

The companies building those interfaces are positioned to lead the largest physiological-health transformation of the digital era. The framework, the science, the practice, and the partnership invitation are all in the book this appendix sits inside.

The Workforce-Health Case

A practical first step for any organization is to make vitality measurable: Invite your team to take their Vitality Score—a simple, private four-part self-assessment of energy, focus, sleep, and presence—on day one and again thirty days later. It turns an abstract benefit into a number a leader can see move.

Knowledge workers in screen-dependent roles—which now describes the majority of the workforce at any technology company—operate with a sustained postural and respiratory compromise that produces measurable downstream effects on cognitive performance, recovery, and engagement. The research is consistent: Workforce sedentary behavior and sustained postural load are associated with productivity losses estimated at $2,000 per employee per year in published studies. For a three-thousand-person organization, that is $6 million per year in invisible cost—substantially exceeding the cost of any reasonable workforce-physiology intervention.

A modest investment in the framework described in this book—book purchase for every employee, monitor-at-eye-level requirement with company-provided monitor stands, sixty-second physiological alignment at the start of meetings longer than thirty minutes, and a partnership with a Human Doctor for on-site or near-site availability—costs in the range of $100 to $300 per employee in year one and produces measurable returns on workforce vitality metrics within ninety days. The ROI math is favorable across virtually every workforce-size scenario.

The companies that move first on this will set the workforce-vitality standard for their industries. The companies that wait will be explaining, three to five years from now, why their workforce health metrics lag the competitors who moved.

One more argument worth naming for the technology-leader audience. The painkiller economy—the combined market for over-the-counter and prescription pain management, measured in tens of billions of dollars annually in the United States alone—is a market that exists because the population has been trained to respond to signals by suppressing them. Every employee your organization covers through health insurance is a participant in that economy to some degree. The opioid crisis, which has produced one of the largest public health catastrophes in modern American history, is the most visible expression of the paradigm, but it is not the only expression.

Musculoskeletal pain management, chronic headache medication, sleep aids, anti-inflammatories, and the cascading downstream treatments for conditions that began as ignored whispers—all of these are expressions of the same paradigm, all of them are absorbed into employer health costs, and all of them are reducible through the adoption of the pain detector framework this book describes. The workforce that practices PAIN consumes less of the painkiller economy.

The organization that builds its wellness program around pain detection rather than pain suppression reduces its medical claims, its absenteeism, its opioid-related disability exposure, and its cumulative healthcare spend. The financial argument is not controversial. It is not even difficult. It is simply one that the conventional healthcare procurement conversation has not yet been trained to ask.

A little PAIN now can save you a lot of pain later. The organizations that internalize this, at scale, across their workforces—the companies, the schools, the healthcare systems—will define workforce vitality for the decade ahead.

The Product-Design Case

The framework in this book provides specific design principles for the next generation of computing interfaces—principles that point toward products users will engage with at lower physiological cost and that will, over time, generate the trust and loyalty that defines category leadership. The seven design principles articulated in chapter 12 (heads-up default posture, peripheral information density, voice-first interaction, body-reading rather than only behavior-reading, rest-recommending capability, stricter standards for children's devices, and biometric data sovereignty) are the starting framework. The signal-intervention map in chapter 13 is the operational layer. Both are offered in the spirit of partnership.

Any product team that wants to engage more deeply with the framework—through clinical advisory, design consultation, validation studies of specific interventions, or co-development of physiologically informed product features—should consider this appendix the open invitation. The authors are available. The framework is documented. The willingness to collaborate is genuine.

The Partnership Case

The Look Up movement is being built as a multi-stakeholder framework, not a single-company or single-profession initiative. Partnerships with technology companies—for product co-development, for workforce-health programs, for content licensing, for advisory engagements, for shared research initiatives—are how the framework reaches the scale at which its impact becomes culturally consequential.

Specific partnership categories the authors are actively developing include: product advisory engagements with companies building heads-up computing devices, biometric wearables, AI coaching platforms, or workforce wellness products; workforce wellness program development with employers who want to implement the Human Doctor model, the workplace adaptations described in chapter 8, or custom variations calibrated to their specific workforce demographics and operational realities; content licensing for inclusion in employee onboarding programs, executive education curricula, parent education programs, school health curricula, and healthcare practitioner continuing education; research partnerships for clinical or workplace validation of specific interventions, particularly when the partner organization has the data infrastructure to support the validation work and the research interest to publish the findings; and speaking and keynote engagements at industry conferences, internal company events, and educational institutions where the framework needs to reach decision-makers in person.

How to Begin

The lowest-friction first step is internal: Read the book, identify the people in your organization who would most benefit from engagement with the framework, and convene a thirty-minute conversation about what application would look like in your specific context. The framework is robust enough to support a wide variety of applications and modest enough to begin with operational simplicity rather than transformational complexity.

The second step, when you are ready for it, is contact. The authors are reachable through the book's website (lookupthebook.com) and respond to qualified partnership inquiries within a working week. The Human Doctor Institute maintains a practitioner directory and a curriculum infrastructure that can be adapted to organizational deployments at most scales.

What an Early-Adopter Organization Looks Like

Imagine a mid-market software company—three hundred employees, distributed-first, the kind of organization in which the average employee spends nine to eleven hours per day in front of a screen and most of the leadership team has personally felt the cumulative cost. Call them, for the purpose of illustration, Northstar Analytics. Northstar is a composite, drawn from the kinds of organizations that have begun moving in this direction.

Northstar's VP of People is reading this book on a flight in late spring. She underlines the chapter on workplace physiology. She lands at her destination, opens her laptop in the airport lounge, and writes a memo to her CEO that begins: "I think I have just read the document that describes what has been happening to our workforce, and I think there is a tractable response."

Within thirty days, Northstar has done four things. First, every employee has received a copy of the book and a Friday-afternoon hour blocked on their calendar to read the first three chapters together as a company-wide initiative. Second, the company has piloted a "monitor-at-eye-level" requirement for everyone working from a primary workstation, with the company providing monitor stands to anyone who needs them—total cost, $4,200, less than half of one developer's monthly salary. Third, every meeting longer than thirty minutes now begins with sixty seconds of physiological alignment, modeled by the most senior person in the room. The cue is deliberately simple: Someone says, "Let's take twenty seconds," and the whole room pauses, pays attention inside now, and does the Lift together—a shared signal that everyone is bringing their most present, regulated, fully alive self to what follows. Fourth, the company has partnered with a chiropractor trained in the Human Doctor model who comes to the headquarters one day a week and is available to every employee for a fifteen-minute spinal assessment and adjustment as a benefit, with sessions booked through the same internal scheduling tool that handles meeting rooms.

Six months later, the company's anonymous quarterly employee survey shows the highest scores on the "energy at end of day" and "ability to focus during deep work blocks" questions in the company's history. Health-insurance utilization for musculoskeletal complaints is down 22 percent. The VP of People presents the data at the company's all-hands meeting and the CEO uses it as the lead example in his next investor update. Two competitors hear about the program through industry channels and begin similar initiatives. The company's recruiting page now features the program as a benefit. Three engineering candidates have cited it as a factor in accepting offers.

None of this required a regulatory change. None of it required platform redesign. None of it required new technology. It required a leadership team that read a book, took the framework seriously, and built four small operational decisions around it. The framework was here. The willingness was the variable.

This is what early adoption looks like at the organizational scale. It is unspectacular. It is operationally simple. It compounds rapidly. And it is available, beginning Monday morning, to every leadership team that decides their workforce's physiological capacity is worth the modest investment of attention and resources required to support it. The companies that move first will define what workforce vitality looks like in their industry. The companies that wait will be explaining, five years from now, why their workforce health metrics lag the competitors who moved.

> The heads-up future will be built. The question is who builds it, with what framework guiding the decisions that will shape what billions of human bodies experience over the next two decades. The framework in this book is one contribution to that work. The collaboration we are inviting is the next.

APPENDIX C

A Reading Group Guide

A little PAIN now can save you a lot of pain later. Hold that sentence through the discussion that follows—it is the argument of the book in eleven words, and each of these questions is an invitation to test it against your own life.

The following questions are designed for book clubs, organizational reading groups, classroom use, and anyone who wants to go deeper into the ideas in *Look Up*. They are organized by chapter and by theme. Use them selectively—not every group will want to cover every chapter, and the thematic questions at the end are designed to work as stand-alone conversations without requiring the chapter-by-chapter discussion.

One recommendation before you begin: Do the Twenty-Second Lift at the start of your reading group session. Not as a demonstration—as a practice. Twenty seconds, practiced together, before any discussion. Notice what changes. That noticing is, in many ways, the best possible entry point into everything the book is trying to say.

By Chapter

Introduction and Chapter 1

- Before you read the sixty-pound number, did you have any awareness of the postural demands of your screen use? How did that number land when you encountered it?
- The book describes Tech Posture Syndrome as a design problem rather than an individual failure. Do you find that framing more or less motivating than a personal health framing? Why?
- Take a lateral posture photograph of yourself as the chapter 1 Put It into Practice section suggests. What do you see? What does it feel like to see it?

- Daniel Ruiz describes himself as "thirty percent less effective" before his posture photograph. Can you identify what percentage of yourself you might currently be giving to the work and relationships in your life?

Chapters 2 and 3

- The children chapter is placed second deliberately—the book argues that protecting a child is often more motivating than protecting oneself. Is that true for you?
- The skull bone study describes children's skeletons reshaping in response to device posture. What is your emotional response to that finding? What, if anything, does it change about how you think about your children's screen use?
- Of the four costs described in chapter 3—physical, cognitive, emotional, and relational—which is most recognizable in your own life? Which would you most want to address first?
- The book describes the "half presence at your own dinner table" as the most intimate cost of Tech Posture Syndrome. Have you experienced this, either as the person giving half presence or as the person receiving it?

Chapters 4 and 5

- The state chain—environment to posture to breath to nervous system state to behavior to outcomes—runs in reverse. Which link in the chain feels most actionable to you? Where would you most naturally intervene?
- The sensory diet audit asks you to rate seven inputs on a scale of one to ten. Which of your inputs is lowest? What would it take to raise it by two points?
- The reframe from "exercise program" to "feeding program" changes the emotional relationship to the practices. Does it change yours? How?
- The book argues that your anxiety may be a breath—not a thought. Does that reframe change anything about how you relate to anxiety in your own life?

Chapters 6 through 9

- Sophia Jones says she is "done needing to understand it. It works." Where in your life do you find yourself waiting to fully understand something before you will try it? Is there a Twenty-Second Lift equivalent—a small practice you could try before you fully understand why?
- The Look Up Day architecture—morning alignment, trigger-paired Lifts, movement snacks, evening alignment—assumes an ordinary workday. How

would you adapt it to your actual life? What is the minimum version that would still be meaningful?

- The threshold practice—twenty seconds of physiological preparation before engaging with someone you love—is the simplest intervention in the book. Have you tried it? What happened?
- Elena spent two minutes in the car before going inside, and her child noticed within five minutes. What does that speed of recognition tell you about children's sensitivity to parental physiological state?

Chapters 10 through 13

- The book argues that medicine is not failing—it is succeeding at what it was designed for, which is not the same as what we need it to do. Do you find this distinction convincing? What would a healthcare system designed for vitality rather than pathology look like in your community?
- The Human Doctor model asks, "What are you capable of?" rather than "What is wrong with you?" Have you ever had a clinician ask you the first question? What would it mean to find one who did?
- Marcus adopted heads-up computing for efficiency reasons and discovered a physiological benefit he hadn't sought. Can you identify other technology or lifestyle choices you have made that have had unexpected physiological effects—positive or negative?
- The distinction between biometric tracking (rearview mirror) and functional support technology (navigation) is central to chapter 13. How do you currently use the health data you track? Are you keeping score or building a feedback loop?
- The book describes the painkiller paradigm versus the pain detector paradigm as two different theories of health. Think about the most recent time you took an over-the-counter painkiller or considered taking one. What was the whisper the body was sending? What would responding to the whisper directly—rather than suppressing it—have looked like? Where in your life has the painkiller paradigm been running without your conscious examination?

Chapters 14 and 15

- The compound interest metaphor runs through chapter 14. Where else in your life have you experienced the return on consistent small inputs? What made the consistency possible?
- The book argues that the physiological state in which much of the population spends most of its waking hours is not the state from which good

collective reasoning proceeds. Do you find the connection between personal physiology and social/political quality compelling? Where do you agree and where do you push back?

- The two futures described in chapter 15—one organized around algorithmic compliance, one around human vitality—are both being built right now. Which do you see more evidence of in your own life, workplace, and community?
- The Power of One closing argues that each regulated nervous system ripples outward through every relationship it inhabits. Can you identify one relationship in your life where this has been true—where one person's physiological state changed the quality of a shared experience?

Thematic Questions

On Technology and the Body

- The book frames the Heads-Down World as a design problem, not a technology problem. Is there a meaningful difference? Who should be responsible for addressing the physiological consequences of technology design?
- Marcus's Ray-Ban and Oakley glasses deliver physiological benefit as a by-product of a technology choice made for efficiency reasons. Is that the right model—embedding health benefits in products people adopt for other reasons? Or is there something important lost when health becomes a side effect rather than a deliberate choice?
- The book predicts that Human Doctors will begin recommending heads-up computing devices as clinical tools, the way medical doctors prescribe pharmaceuticals. What would it take for that to become standard practice? What barriers exist?

On Healthcare and Vitality

- The book is explicit that it is "not anti-medicine, but pro-vitality." Do you find that distinction clear and meaningful? Where does medicine end and vitality care begin in your own experience?
- The *Gattaca* analogy describes a future in which biometric compliance determines medical status. Do you see evidence of this direction in current healthcare? Is it inevitable? Is it avoidable?
- The book argues that the largest unrealized economic return available to any organization is the elimination of the cognitive cost of Tech Posture Syndrome in its workforce. If you are an organizational leader, what would it take to make that argument persuasively to your board or investors?

On the Civilizational Argument

- The Society That Looks Up section connects personal physiological dysregulation to the quality of civic and political life. How much of the current social and political chaos do you think is physiological in origin? How much do you think is addressable through the practices in this book?
- The compound interest of collective vitality—millions of regulated nervous systems, rippling outward—is the book's most ambitious claim. Is it too ambitious? Or is it not ambitious enough?
- If you could change one thing in your community, your organization, or your family based on what you have read in this book, what would it be? And what is the smallest possible first step toward that change?

For additional discussion resources, practitioner guides, and the complete Look Up Challenge community, visit lookupthebook.com.

APPENDIX D

The First Thirty Days

A Day-by-Day Framework

This appendix provides a day-by-day framework for the first thirty days of Look Up practice. Each day has one focus—one thing to add, refine, or deepen—so that the full protocol is built gradually, one layer at a time, without the overwhelming detail that causes most wellness programs to collapse.

The goal of thirty days is not completion. It is momentum. By day thirty, you will have practiced the core elements enough times that they have begun to feel less like a program and more like a life. That shift—from doing to being—is the destination.

A note on imperfection: Miss a day and pick up where you left off. The practice is not damaged by gaps. It is built by returns.

Week 1: Foundation—The Twenty-Second Lift

Day 1: Take your lateral posture photograph. Practice the Twenty-Second Lift three times today—morning, midday, evening. Note your starting state in a single sentence: How do I feel right now, physically and mentally?

Day 2: Choose your first trigger pairing. One thing you do every day without exception. Attach the Lift to it. Every single time, without exception, for the rest of the challenge.

Day 3: Raise your monitor to eye level. Measure, adjust, and work from this height for the rest of the challenge.

Day 4: Add a second trigger pairing. Two consistent Lift triggers now in place.

Day 5: Practice the physiological sigh three times today—at moments of elevated stress or low energy. Double inhale through the nose, long exhale through the mouth. Notice the immediate effect.

Day 6: Add a third trigger pairing. Three triggers attached. The Lift should now be happening, on average, ten to fifteen times per day without requiring you to remember it independently.

Day 7: Week 1 review. How many Lifts did you do? What changed in your body? What did you notice in your state after each one? Adjust your trigger pairings if they are not firing reliably.

Week 2: Morning and Evening

Day 8: Implement the morning alignment for the first time. Breathe before you screen. Ten full breaths at the edge of the bed. Two minutes of spinal movement. Far-gaze for thirty seconds. Then begin your day.

Day 9: Implement the evening alignment. Screen away fifteen minutes before sleep. Two minutes on the floor, ten slow breaths. One acknowledgment.

Day 10: Practice both alignments. Begin tracking your sleep quality this week—not the number, but the subjective sense of restoration.

Day 11: Add your first scheduled movement snack—at the ninety-minute mark of your primary work block. Stand, extend, rotate, side-bend. One minute.

Day 12: Add a second movement snack. Two movement breaks now in the workday, separated by approximately ninety minutes.

Day 13: Practice the regulation breath (four counts in, eight counts out) for five minutes before your most challenging interaction of the day.

Day 14: Week 2 review. Morning alignment, evening alignment, two movement snacks, three trigger-paired Lifts. How is your sleep? Your afternoon energy? The quality of your presence when you arrive home?

Week 3: Work and Relationships

Day 15: Implement state-based scheduling. Identify your two highest-quality hours. Protect them for your most demanding cognitive work. Move administrative and reactive tasks to lower-energy periods.

Day 16: Begin the forty-five-minute movement interval rule. Set an alarm. Every forty-five minutes, stand and do the Lift. No exceptions today.

Day 17: Practice the threshold before one significant relationship interaction today. Twenty seconds before you walk through the door, sit at the table, or answer the phone.

Day 18: Practice the far-gaze break three times today—thirty to sixty seconds of looking away from all screens, eyes soft, peripheral field active.

Day 19: Practice the full Look Up Ritual (the extended version from chapter 6) once today—five minutes, full sequence.

Day 20: Threshold practice for every significant relationship interaction today. Not just one—all of them.

Day 21: Week 3 review. What has changed in your work quality? In your relationships? In your energy at the end of the day? Write one sentence for each domain.

Week 4: Integration and Identity

Day 22: Conduct your sensory diet audit from chapter 5. Rate all seven inputs on a scale of one to ten. Identify the most depleted. Add one targeted practice today.

Day 23: Practice the activation breath in the morning. Note its effect on your starting state compared to your Day 1 baseline.

Day 23.5 (Pain Detector Day): Choose one persistent physical signal in your body—a tightness, an ache, a chronic low-grade discomfort you have been managing with a painkiller, a stretch, a workaround, or simple avoidance. Instead of suppressing it today, pay attention to it. Notice when it intensifies and when it eases. Notice what preceded each change. Notice what the body is telling you through this signal that you have not fully received. Do not act on the information yet. Just receive it. Tomorrow, decide what to do with what you learned. This is the practice of being a pain detector rather than a painkiller.

Day 24: Teach someone in your life one element of the Look Up practice. Not the whole book—one thing. The physiological sigh. The morning alignment. The threshold practice. Teaching deepens understanding.

Day 25: Full Look Up Day. Use every element from chapter 7. Morning alignment, trigger-paired Lifts, movement intervals, far-gaze breaks, state-based scheduling, threshold practices, evening alignment.

Day 26: Take your second lateral posture photograph. Compare to Day 1. Note what has changed—in the photograph and in your body's experience of itself.

Day 27: Write your twelve-month projection. Three specific expectations for what consistent practice will produce. Put them somewhere you will find them in a year.

Day 28: Rest from deliberate practice—but maintain your trigger pairings. Notice whether the Lifts happen automatically now, without the triggers needing to prompt them. That automaticity is identity in formation.

Day 29: Identify one structural environmental change to support long-term practice—a workspace adjustment, a schedule change, a relationship commitment, a new trigger. Implement it today.

Day 30: Full review. Compare your state today to Day 1. What has changed? What is still developing? What do you want to build in month two? Write it down. The challenge ends. The practice continues.

The 30-Day Challenge is not the destination. It is the on-ramp. By day thirty, you have built the habits, seen the evidence in your own body, and begun to understand what the practice gives you. What follows is simply living it—for a month, then a year, then a decade, then a lifetime of compound returns on the direction you chose to look.

APPENDIX E

A Note on the Science

This book is written for a general readership with the voice of accessible confidence that the strength of the underlying evidence warrants. It draws on peer-reviewed research in biomechanics, neuroscience, respiratory physiology, occupational health, behavioral psychology, longevity science, and polyvagal theory.

Where findings are preliminary or contested, we have tried to say so. Where the evidence is robust and converging across multiple research traditions, we have presented it with the confidence it deserves. We are practitioners, not academics, and we write with the perspective of people who have watched this science change the lives of the patients we have served across a combined half century of clinical work.

The research told us why. Our patients showed us that it was true.

The Notes and Bibliography that follow provide the primary sources for specific claims throughout the text. Readers wishing to investigate the underlying science are encouraged to start there.

APPENDIX F

For Practitioners

Clinical Integration Notes

The following notes were integrated throughout the main text in earlier drafts of this book. We have consolidated them here so clinical readers can access the practitioner-focused material in one place, and so the main text flows more naturally for the general reader.

The clinical framework offered here is practical, not prescriptive. The four notes below address the sensory diet, the Look Up Day protocol, the workplace clinical encounter, and the relational prescription. Adapt any of them to the patient population, practice model, and clinical scope you are working in. The shared goal is to move Tech Posture Syndrome from an unnamed pattern your patients present with to a nameable, addressable clinical focus with specific, documentable interventions and measurable outcomes.

A little PAIN now can save you a lot of pain later. The practitioners who teach this to their patients—and who model the practice in their own bodies—are the clinical anchors of the movement this book describes.

Note 1: The Sensory Diet Assessment

The sensory diet framework gives practitioners a clinical lens for a category of patient complaint that has no standard diagnostic code: the diffuse underperformance of a nervous system that is physiologically deficient in the inputs it requires. The seven-item sensory diet audit in this chapter is a reliable clinical screening. Patients who score below three in four or more categories are, in our clinical experience, presenting with nervous system dysregulation driven primarily by environmental deprivation rather than structural pathology, and their care plan should address the environmental inputs as explicitly as it addresses the structural findings.

The highest-yield clinical intervention for sensory diet deficiency is the prescription of specific environmental changes rather than additional in-office treatment alone. A patient who understands that their fatigue is a sensory nutrition deficiency and who can identify the specific inputs that are lowest will make environmental changes more consistently than a patient who has been given exercises to perform. The reframing from "What is wrong with your body?" to "What does your nervous system need that it has not been getting?" is itself a therapeutic intervention—it shifts the patient from passive recipient to active participant in their own restoration.

Note 2: Prescribing the Look Up Day

The Look Up Day architecture is most effectively introduced to patients as a prescription in the literal sense: a specific recommendation, written in the chart, with specific elements and specific expected outcomes that will be reviewed at the next appointment. The components that produce the highest clinical return when added sequentially are, in order of priority: first, the morning alignment (breathe before screen); second, the evening alignment (screen away, floor position, one acknowledgment); third, the movement snack schedule; and fourth, the trigger-paired Lifts.

The sequence matters because each element builds the physiological foundation for the next. Morning alignment sets the neurological baseline. Evening alignment sets the conditions for restorative sleep, which improves the quality of the next morning's baseline. Movement snacks prevent the accumulation that erodes the gains of morning and evening. The Lifts distribute corrections throughout the day. Introduce them in this order, with a two-week practice window for each before adding the next, and the clinical return will be substantially higher than introducing all elements simultaneously.

Note 3: Bringing the Look Up Practice into the Clinic

The workplace chapters of this book are relevant to every practitioner whose patients spend significant time in knowledge-work environments—which, in the current economy, is most of them. The following clinical framework supports the integration of workplace assessment and intervention into your existing practice model.

The workplace assessment begins with three questions that most clinicians never ask and that patients, in our experience, almost always find illuminating:

- How many hours per day do you spend looking at a screen?
- What is your monitor height relative to your eyes?
- Do you have any scheduled breaks from sustained screen engagement?

The answers to these three questions will, in a significant proportion of your patients, identify the primary environmental driver of the physiological pattern you are treating.

The highest-yield clinical recommendation for most knowledge workers is the monitor height adjustment. It is free, it is immediate, and it produces continuous postural improvement for every hour the patient is at their desk—without requiring any ongoing attention or willpower. After establishing a neutral head position in your examination, show the patient what their ear-over-shoulder alignment looks like and instruct them to bring their monitor to the height that allows them to maintain that alignment while working. Follow up at the next visit with a brief postural assessment to confirm the adjustment has been made.

The trigger-pairing recommendation is the second-highest yield. Identify two or three actions the patient performs without exception every day—answering a phone call, sitting down at their desk, finishing a meeting. Pair the Twenty-Second Lift explicitly with each trigger. Write it in the chart. Review it at the next visit. The patient who has the Lift paired to triggers they already execute does not need to find time for a new habit. They are executing the habit at moments they would have executed the trigger anyway.

Finally: Normalize workplace practice as clinical care. Many patients hesitate to take movement breaks or practice postural correction at work because the culture of their workplace equates stillness with productivity. Clinician recommendation carries specific authority in this context. "My doctor said I should do this" is a social permission structure that makes behavior in a workplace culture context significantly easier. Use it. Recommend the Twenty-Second Lift explicitly, document the recommendation, and ask the patient at every visit how consistently they are executing it. The documentation creates accountability. The accountability creates compliance. The compliance creates the compound return that is the point of the entire protocol.

Note 4: The Relational Prescription

The threshold practice is the most immediately impactful relational intervention available through the Look Up Practice, and it is the one that most patients will not think to do without explicit clinical recommendation. The prescription is specific: Before engaging with any person whose presence deserves your best—entering your home, sitting down to a meal, beginning a phone call with someone you love—perform the Twenty-Second Lift. The specificity of the prescription (this practice, at this moment, for this purpose) is what makes it clinically effective rather than a vague aspiration.

In the chart, record the threshold practice as a relational prescription alongside the structural and movement recommendations. At the next visit, ask specifically:

- Are you doing it?
- When?
- What are you noticing/feeling?

APPENDIX G

Words We Have Redefined

A Short Glossary

Good books change how readers use certain words. Great books do it on purpose. This short glossary names the words this book is using in a way that may differ from the reader's default understanding and gives each term the specific meaning that makes the book's argument coherent. Keep this page. Reference it when any of these words appears in your reading, in your conversations, or in your own body.

Adjustment. Not only a clinical procedure. Every breath is an adjustment. Every thought. Every choice. Every moment of paying attention inside now. The body adjusts automatically, the mind adjusts automatically, and the awareness adjusts by choice. The skilled hands-on adjustment a Human Doctor performs is one valuable form of a universal activity that every living system is already performing, continuously, as the literal definition of being alive. Adjustments are great things. Make them well. Make them often.

Health. Not the absence of disease, but the presence of vitality. Not what your blood work does not show, but what your nervous system does express when it is given the inputs it requires. Health is not a score. Health is a capacity—to adapt, to recover, to be fully alive in the body you are inhabiting.

Healthcare. Not what happens when something goes wrong. What happens in the continuous, proactive tending of the nervous system and the body it coordinates. A healthcare system organized around reactive disease management is what we currently have. A healthcare system organized around proactive vitality is what the framework of this book makes possible.

Human Doctor. A practitioner who centers the nervous system, who supports Innate Intelligence rather than overriding it, and whose clinical practice is organized around the Tune-In and Tune-Up rather than around disease management and symptom suppression. The Human Doctor model is described in detail in chapter 11. It is the clinical form of the practice that the rest of the book teaches in personal form.

Intelligence. Not only what happens in a brain. Universal Intelligence is the organizing principle of the larger order in which life exists. Innate Intelligence is the local expression of that order in the form of your body—the continuous self-organizing activity that keeps you alive without your conscious involvement. Artificial intelligence is the engineered intelligence built by humans. Three intelligences. Held in the right order, a life of coherence. Held in the wrong order, the cost that much of this book has been documenting.

Look Up. A physical practice, a daily discipline, a philosophical orientation, and an invitation. Physically: the cervical extension and gaze elevation that reverses the load of the Heads-Down World on the human nervous system. Daily: the many small moments of PAIN and the Twenty-Second Lift that accumulate into a life of vitality. Philosophically: the choice to inhabit your body fully, rather than surrender it to the interface the Heads-Down World has been designing around. As an invitation: the movement this book is building.

A little PAIN now can save you a lot of pain later. Hold that. Take it with you. Redefine the words you thought you knew and notice what changes in the body that has been carrying you through a life you have not yet fully inhabited. The rest of the practice is available to you, every breath, starting now.

Pain. Not an enemy to be eliminated, but information to be received. The body's notification system—a whisper at first, a scream only when the whisper has been ignored long enough. The cultural treatment of pain as the problem has generated a trillion-dollar healthcare cascade and an opioid crisis. This book treats pain as the signal.

PAIN (the practice). Pay attention inside now. The practice at the center of this book. A thought process first and a physical practice second—the discipline of receiving the body's signals rather than suppressing them. PAIN is the practice that turns a person from a painkiller into a pain detector, and it is the practice that makes every other practice in this book work.

Pain detector. The inverse of painkiller. A person whose default response to a body signal is to receive it and respond with the input the body is asking for, rather than suppress it. Every human body is already a pain detector; the practice of PAIN is how a person becomes consciously available to what their detector has been telling them all along.

Painkiller. Two meanings. The narrow meaning: an over-the-counter or prescription medication that suppresses a pain signal without addressing its cause. The broader meaning: any orientation—pharmaceutical, behavioral, cultural—that treats a body signal as something to be silenced rather than received. The painkiller paradigm, taken at population scale, is the engine of much of what is failing in modern healthcare.

Tune-In and Tune-Up. The ritual of proactive physiological maintenance performed with a skilled Human Doctor. The tune-in is the clinical form of PAIN—paying attention, inside, now, with a trained practitioner as your guide. The tune-up is what the practitioner's skilled hands do with what the tune-in reveals. Together, they are the clinical complement to the personal daily practice of the Twenty-Second Lift.

Bibliography

Organized by chapter. For a complete reference list, visit lookupthebook.com.

Introduction and Chapters 1–4

Hansraj, Kenneth K. "Assessment of Stresses in the Cervical Spine Caused by Posture and Position of the Head." *Surgical Technology International* 25 (2014): 277–79.

Damasceno, Gabriela M., et al. "Text Neck and Neck Pain in 18–21-Year-Old Young Adults." *European Spine Journal* 27, no. 6 (2018): 1249–54. doi.org/10.1007/s00586-017-5444-5.

Shahar, David, and Mark G. L. Sayers. "Prominent Exostosis Projecting from the Occipital Squama More Substantial and Prevalent in Young Adult than Older Age Groups." *Scientific Reports* 8 (2018): art. 3354. doi.org/10.1038/s41598-018-21625-1. See also the Author Correction, *Scientific Reports* 9 (2019): art. 13707.

Twenge, Jean M., et al. "Increases in Depressive Symptoms, Suicide-Related Outcomes, and Suicide Rates among US Adolescents after 2010 and Links to Increased New Media Screen Time." *Clinical Psychological Science* 6, no. 1 (2018): 3–17. doi.org/10.1177/2167702617723376.

Haidt, Jonathan, and Jean Twenge. "Is There an Increase in Adolescent Mood Disorders, Self-Harm, and Suicide since 2010 in the USA and UK?" *Emotion Review* 13, no. 1 (2021). doi.org/10.1177/1754073920982890.

Nair, Shwetha, et al. "Do Slumped and Upright Postures Affect Stress Responses? A Randomized Trial." *Health Psychology* 34, no. 6 (2015): 632–41. doi.org/10.1037/hea0000146.

Thayer, Julian F., Fredrik Åhs, Mats Fredrikson, John J. Sollers III, and Tor D. Wager. "A Meta-analysis of Heart Rate Variability and Neuroimaging Studies: Implications for Heart Rate Variability as a Marker of Stress and

Health." *Neuroscience & Biobehavioral Reviews* 36, no. 2 (2012): 747–56. doi.org/10.1016/j.neubiorev.2011.11.009.

Barrett, Lisa Feldman. *How Emotions Are Made: The Secret Life of the Brain*. Boston: Houghton Mifflin Harcourt, 2017.

Carney, Dana R., Amy J. C. Cuddy, and Andy J. Yap. "Power Posing: Brief Nonverbal Displays Affect Neuroendocrine Levels and Risk Tolerance." *Psychological Science* 21, no. 10 (2010): 1363–68. doi.org/10.1177/0956797610383437. The hormonal findings did not replicate; see Ranehill et al., "Assessing the Robustness of Power Posing," *Psychological Science* 26, no. 5 (2015): 653–56, doi.org/10.1177/0956797614553946.

Patel, Hemal H., et al. "Neural and Molecular Changes during a Mind-Body Reconceptualization, Meditation, and Open-Label Placebo Healing Intervention." *Communications Biology* 8 (2025): art. 1525. doi.org/10.1038/s42003-025-08846-7.

Stapleton, Peta, Joe Dispenza, et al. "Large Effects of Brief Meditation Intervention on EEG Spectra in Meditation Novices." *Brain and Behavior* 10, no. 11 (2020): art. e2900. doi.org/10.1002/brb3.2900.

Peper, Erik, and I-Mei Lin. "Increase or Decrease Depression: How Body Postures Influence Your Energy Level." *Biofeedback* 40, no. 3 (2012): 92–96. doi.org/10.5298/1081-5937-40.3.01.

Cuddy, Amy J. C., Caroline A. Wilmuth, Andy J. Yap, and Dana R. Carney. "Preparatory Power Posing Affects Nonverbal Presence and Job Interview Performance." *Journal of Applied Psychology* 100, no. 4 (2015): 1286–95. doi.org/10.1037/a0038543.

Chapters 5–9

Porges, Stephen W. *The Polyvagal Theory: Neurophysiological Foundations of Emotions, Attachment, Communication, and Self-Regulation*. New York: W. W. Norton, 2011.

Ashhad, Sufyan, Kaitlyn Kam, Christopher A. Del Negro, and Jack L. Feldman. "Breathing Rhythm and Pattern and Their Influence on Emotion." *Annual Review of Neuroscience* 45 (2022): 223–47. doi.org/10.1146/annurev-neuro-090121-014424.

Thayer, Julian F., et al. "A Meta-analysis of Heart Rate Variability and Neuroimaging Studies." *Neuroscience & Biobehavioral Reviews* 36, no. 2 (2012): 747–56. doi.org/10.1016/j.neubiorev.2011.11.009.

Clear, James. *Atomic Habits: An Easy and Proven Way to Build Good Habits and Break Bad Ones*. New York: Avery, 2018.

Fogg, BJ. *Tiny Habits: The Small Changes That Change Everything.* Boston: Houghton Mifflin Harcourt, 2019.

Wood, Wendy, and David T. Neal. "A New Look at Habits and the Habit-Goal Interface." *Psychological Review* 114, no. 4 (2007): 843–63. doi.org/10.1037/0033-295X.114.4.843.

Biswas, Aviroop, et al. "Sedentary Time and Its Association with Risk for Disease Incidence, Mortality, and Hospitalization in Adults." *Annals of Internal Medicine* 162, no. 2 (2015): 123–32. doi.org/10.7326/M14-1651.

Garber, Carol Ewing, et al. "American College of Sports Medicine Position Stand: Quantity and Quality of Exercise for Developing and Maintaining Cardiorespiratory, Musculoskeletal, and Neuromotor Fitness in Apparently Healthy Adults." *Medicine & Science in Sports & Exercise* 43, no. 7 (2011): 1334–59. doi.org/10.1249/MSS.0b013e318213fefb.

Chapters 10–13

Porges, Stephen W. *The Polyvagal Theory.* New York: W. W. Norton, 2011.

Rubinstein, Sidney M., et al. "Spinal Manipulative Therapy for Chronic Low-Back Pain." *Cochrane Database of Systematic Reviews,* no. 2 (2011): CD008112. doi.org/10.1002/14651858.CD008112.pub2.

Fries, James F. "Aging, Natural Death, and the Compression of Morbidity." *New England Journal of Medicine* 303, no. 3 (1980): 130–35. doi.org/10.1056/NEJM198007173030304.

Hyman, Mark. *Young Forever: The Secrets to Living Your Longest, Healthiest Life.* New York: Little, Brown Spark, 2023.

World Health Organization. "Burn-out an 'Occupational Phenomenon': International Classification of Diseases." May 28, 2019. who.int/news/item/28-05-2019-burn-out-an-occupational-phenomenon-international-classification-of-diseases.

Health Enhancement Research Organization. *HERO Research Study: Employee Health & Productivity.* 2019. hero-health.org.

Chapters 14–15 and Appendices

Clear, James. *Atomic Habits.* New York: Avery, 2018.

Duhigg, Charles. *The Power of Habit: Why We Do What We Do in Life and Business.* New York: Random House, 2012.

Chomitz, Virginia R., et al. "Is There a Relationship between Physical Fitness and Academic Achievement? Positive Results from Public School Children in the Northeastern United States." *Journal of School Health* 79, no. 1 (2009): 30–37. doi.org/10.1111/j.1746-1561.2008.00371.x.

Benden, Mark E., et al. "The Impact of Stand-Biased Desks in Classrooms on Calorie Expenditure in Children." *American Journal of Public Health* 101, no. 8 (2011): 1433–36. doi.org/10.2105/AJPH.2010.300072.

Pink, Daniel H. *Drive: The Surprising Truth about What Motivates Us*. New York: Riverhead Books, 2009.

Haavik, Heidi, and Bernadette Murphy. "The Role of Spinal Manipulation in Addressing Disordered Sensorimotor Integration and Altered Motor Control." *Journal of Electromyography and Kinesiology* 22, no. 5 (2012): 768–76. doi.org/10.1016/j.jelekin.2012.02.012.

Taylor, Heidi Haavik, and Bernadette Murphy. "Cervical Spine Manipulation Alters Sensorimotor Integration: A Somatosensory Evoked Potential Study." *Clinical Neurophysiology* 118, no. 2 (2007): 391–402. doi.org/10.1016/j.clinph.2006.09.014.

Haavik, Heidi, et al. "The Contemporary Model of Vertebral Column Joint Dysfunction and Impact of High-Velocity, Low-Amplitude Controlled Vertebral Thrusts on Neuromuscular Function." *European Journal of Applied Physiology* 121, no. 10 (2021): 2675–2720. doi.org/10.1007/s00421-021-04727-z.

Hansraj, Kenneth K. "Assessment of Stresses in the Cervical Spine Caused by Posture and Position of the Head." *Surgical Technology International* 25 (2014): 277–79.

Epel, Elissa S., et al. "More Than a Feeling: A Unified View of Stress Measurement for Population Science." *Frontiers in Neuroendocrinology* 49 (2018): 146–69. doi.org/10.1016/j.yfrne.2018.03.001.

Porges, Stephen W. "Neuroception: A Subconscious System for Detecting Threats and Safety." *Zero to Three* 24, no. 5 (2004): 19–24.

Haidt, Jonathan. *The Anxious Generation: How the Great Rewiring of Childhood Is Causing an Epidemic of Mental Illness*. New York: Penguin Press, 2024.

Ayres, A. Jean. *Sensory Integration and Learning Disorders*. Los Angeles: Western Psychological Services, 1972.

Fries, James F., et al. "Compression of Morbidity 1980–2011: A Focused Review of Paradigms and Progress." *Journal of Aging Research* 2011: art. 261702. doi.org/10.4061/2011/261702.

Laird, Angela R., et al. "Cognitive Neuroscience of Emotional Regulation." *Neuropsychologia* 49, no. 6 (2011): 1346–57. doi.org/10.1016/j.neuropsychologia.2011.02.045.

Dallman, Mary F., et al. "Chronic Stress and Obesity: A New View of 'Comfort Food.'" *Proceedings of the National Academy of Sciences* 100, no. 20 (2003): 11696–701. doi.org/10.1073/pnas.1934666100.

Acknowledgments

A book about the nervous system, written by three people who spent two years in deep conversation about the nervous system, is itself a demonstration of the argument. We are better together than any of us would have been alone. This is where our gratitude begins.

To the patients across three practices and sixty combined years of clinical work: You are in every page of this book, even the ones that do not appear to be about you. Your willingness to share what was happening in your bodies—to say, "I don't know why, but something is off" and to trust us with the answer—is the reason this book exists. The composite characters who carry your stories through these chapters are our attempt to honor the full pattern of what you showed us while protecting the privacy of each of you individually.

To the researchers whose work anchors the science in these pages—Dr. Stephen Porges, Dr. Kenneth Hansraj, Dr. Andrew Huberman, Dr. Amy Cuddy, Dr. Erik Peper, Dr. James Fries, Dr. Heidi Haavik and the many others cited in our bibliography—thank you for doing the rigorous work that makes books like this one defensible. We have tried to represent your findings faithfully. Any errors of interpretation are our own.

To Life University, its leadership, its faculty, its students, and the decades of vitalistic tradition it carries forward: Thank you for being the institutional home of the philosophy this book is built on. The Human Doctor model is not a departure from what Life University has always done. It is its next expression.

To the colleagues, mentors, and fellow practitioners who have shaped how each of us understands the body and its capacity—there are too many to name completely, and the omissions are not oversights but limitations of space. You know who you are. This book carries your fingerprints.

From Gilles: To Melissa, my wife and partner in everything—thank you for being by my side. To my children and grandchildren: You are why I still get up at 5:00 a.m. To my mentor Dr. James W. Parker, who taught me that loving service must be my first technique—I have tried to live up to that my entire career. To my colleagues at Life University, thank you for your constant support. To the Jamaican

Olympian who watched me run and decided I was worth coaching: You changed the last chapter of my story.

From Jeff: To my family, who tolerated the late nights and the early mornings and the constant conversation about nervous systems and posture and what we were trying to say: thank you. To the thousands of practitioners who have engaged with The Evidence Based Chiropractor and The Smart Chiropractor over the years—your questions and your clinical experience shaped what I understand about this work more than any research paper ever could.

From Jason: To the patients and practitioners who have trusted me over the years with their stories and their questions about how to communicate health in a world that makes it so hard to hear—this book is the longest answer I have ever given to the question you kept asking. To my coauthors, Gilles and Jeff, for two years of conversation that sharpened every idea in these pages, and for a friendship that made the work a joy. To the mentors and colleagues across this profession who shaped how I think about the body and its capacity to heal—you taught me that communication is itself an act of care. And to the growing Look Up community—the doctors, leaders, and readers already living this practice and carrying it into their families, their teams, and their world—you are the proof that vitality is contagious.

To my family, who has lived with a person who has been trying to make the case for human vitality since before they can remember: Thank you for believing the case was worth making.

Finally: to everyone who reads this book and looks up—you are the movement. One body at a time. One breath at a time. One Twenty-Second Lift at a time. Take your Vitality Score today. Take it again in thirty days. Then tell someone what changed—because a rising Vitality Score is a story, and shared stories are how a practice becomes a movement.

That is enough. It is more than enough. It is everything.

About the Authors

Dr. Gilles A. LaMarche

Dr. Gilles A. LaMarche is a chiropractor, educator, and author of seventeen books—and the living proof of the central argument of this one. In 2003, at the height of a twenty-five-year clinical career, he was diagnosed with primary pulmonary hypertension and cardiomegaly and given two years to live without surgery. He declined surgery, committed to intensive chiropractic care, and recovered completely. At seventy, he competed at the World Masters Track and Field Championships as a member of Team USA—twenty years after his predicted death.

Dr. LaMarche holds a Bachelor of Science from the University of Toronto and his Doctor of Chiropractic from Canadian Memorial Chiropractic College and is a graduate of the Executive Leadership Program at Cornell University. He serves as Vice President of University Advancement at Life University in Marietta, Georgia—the world's largest chiropractic educational institution—and has lectured on health, vitality, and human performance in more than twenty countries. His personal mission: "I hereby pledge my life to my greatest expression of love and service for the benefit of humanity."

Dr. Jeff Langmaid

Dr. Jeff Langmaid is a serial healthcare entrepreneur, author, and one of the chiropractic profession's most recognized voices on evidence-based practice and health communication. He is the founder of The Evidence Based Chiropractor and cofounder of The Smart Chiropractor, platforms that collectively serve thousands of practices worldwide. His book *Marketing Chiropractic to Medical Doctors* was the number one new release in chiropractic on Amazon; he is also coauthor of *The Payday Practice.*

Dr. Langmaid holds a Bachelor of Science from the University of Tampa and his Doctor of Chiropractic from Palmer College of Chiropractic–Florida. A nationally recognized speaker on research communication and practice innovation, he cohosts the podcast *The Business of Healing* with Dr. Jason A. Deitch.

Dr. Jason A. Deitch

Dr. Jason A. Deitch is a chiropractor, bestselling author, speaker, and health communication strategist who has spent more than three decades helping the science of natural health reach the people who need it most. He believes the future of healthcare is not only what happens in a doctor's office, but what each of us chooses, moment to moment, in the care of our own nervous system. He is coauthor of the bestselling *Discover Wellness: How Staying Healthy Can Make You Rich* and author of *Unmarket Your Practice*, and he was an early pioneer of using social and digital media to carry the message of vitality to a worldwide audience.

As cofounder of The Smart Chiropractor with Dr. Jeff Langmaid, he has helped practitioners around the world communicate the value of proactive care, and his work now focuses on the intersection of human vitality and artificial intelligence—on building the tools, language, and movement to help people everywhere reclaim their health in the age of AI. He is driven by a single conviction: that when people learn to look up, they do not just change their posture—they change the trajectory of their lives.

Dr. Deitch served as Chief Wellness Officer at WellCall, Inc., the nation's leading employer wellness solutions provider. He holds an undergraduate degree in marketing from Northeastern University and his Doctor of Chiropractic from Life University and wrote his first book before attending chiropractic school—a trajectory that signals the driving conviction of his career: that the most important thing in health communication is not what you know, but whether the people who need it can see it, read it, and hear it.

Notes

Chapter 2

1 Shahar D, Sayers MGL. Prominent exostosis projecting from the occipital squama more substantial and prevalent in young adult than older age groups. *Scientific Reports.* 2018;8:3354.

Chapter 3

1 Yong-Hao Pua et al., "Prevalence and Risk Factors Associated with Musculoskeletal Complaints among Users of Mobile Handheld Devices: A Systematic Review," *Applied Ergonomics* 59 (2017): 132–42, doi .org/10.1016/j.apergo.2016.08.020.

Chapter 4

1 Dina Lelic et al., "Manipulation of Dysfunctional Spinal Joints Affects Sensorimotor Integration in the Prefrontal Cortex: A Brain Source Localization Study," *Neural Plasticity* 2016 (2016): art. 3704964, doi .org/10.1155/2016/3704964.

2 Melis Yilmaz Balban et al., "Brief Structured Respiration Practices Enhance Mood and Reduce Physiological Arousal," *Cell Reports Medicine* 4, no. 1 (2023): art. 100895, doi.org/10.1016/j.xcrm.2022.100895.

3 Julian F. Thayer et al., "A Meta-analysis of Heart Rate Variability and Neuroimaging Studies: Implications for Heart Rate Variability as a Marker of Stress and Health," *Neuroscience & Biobehavioral Reviews* 36, no. 2 (2012): 747–56, doi.org/10.1016/j.neubiorev.2011.11.009.

4 Dana R. Carney, Amy J. C. Cuddy, and Andy J. Yap, "Power Posing: Brief Nonverbal Displays Affect Neuroendocrine Levels and Risk Tolerance," *Psychological Science* 21, no. 10 (2010): 1363–68, doi.org /10.1177/0956797610383437. The original neuroendocrine findings did not replicate; see Eva Ranehill et al., "Assessing the Robustness of Power Posing," *Psychological Science* 26, no. 5 (2015): 653–56. For the authors' reanalysis of the broader literature, see Amy J. C. Cuddy, S. Jack Schultz, and Nathan E. Fosse, "P-Curving a More Comprehensive Body of Research on Postural Feedback Reveals Clear Evidential Value for Power-Posing Effects," *Psychological Science* 29, no. 4 (2018): 656–66.

5 Hemal H. Patel et al., "Neural and Molecular Changes during a Mind-Body Reconceptualization, Meditation, and Open-Label Placebo Healing Intervention," *Communications Biology* 8 (2025): art. 1525, doi.org/10.1038/s42003-025-08846-7.

Chapter 5

1 A. Jean Ayres, *Sensory Integration and Learning Disorders* (Los Angeles: Western Psychological Services, 1972).

Chapter 6

1 Paul M. Lehrer and Richard Gevirtz, "Heart Rate Variability Biofeedback: How and Why Does It Work?," *Frontiers in Psychology* 5 (2014): art. 756, doi.org/10.3389/fpsyg.2014.00756.

2 A. D. Craig, "Interoception: The Sense of the Physiological Condition of the Body," *Current Opinion in Neurobiology* 13, no. 4 (2003): 500–505, doi.org/10.1016/S0959-4388(03)00090-4; and A. D. Craig, "How Do You Feel? Interoception: The Sense of the Physiological Condition of the Body," *Nature Reviews Neuroscience* 3, no. 8 (2002): 655–66. See also Hugo D. Critchley and Sarah N. Garfinkel, "Interoception

and Emotion," *Current Opinion in Psychology* 17 (2017): 7–14; and Lisa Feldman Barrett and W. Kyle Simmons, "Interoceptive Predictions in the Brain," *Nature Reviews Neuroscience* 16, no. 7 (2015): 419–29.

3 Tara L. Kraft and Sarah D. Pressman, "Grin and Bear It: The Influence of Manipulated Facial Expression on the Stress Response," *Psychological Science* 23, no. 11 (2012): 1372–78, doi.org/10.1177/0956797612445312. See also Barbara L. Fredrickson and Robert W. Levenson, "Positive Emotions Speed Recovery from the Cardiovascular Sequelae of Negative Emotions," *Cognition & Emotion* 12, no. 2 (1998): 191–220. The broader facial-feedback literature shows mixed replication; the Many Smiles Collaboration, "A Multi-lab Test of the Facial Feedback Hypothesis by the Many Smiles Collaboration," *Nature Human Behaviour* 6 (2022): 1731–42, supports a small but reliable effect.

4 On the minimum-effective-dose framing: brief, repeated autonomic interventions produce measurable shifts in heart-rate variability within one to three breath cycles. See Paul M. Lehrer and Richard Gevirtz, "Heart Rate Variability Biofeedback: How and Why Does It Work?," *Frontiers in Psychology* 5 (2014): art. 756, doi.org/10.3389/fpsyg.2014.00756; and Sylvain Laborde et al., "Effects of Voluntary Slow Breathing on Heart Rate and Heart Rate Variability: A Systematic Review and a Meta-analysis," *Neuroscience & Biobehavioral Reviews* 138 (2022): art. 104711, doi.org/10.1016/j.neubiorev.2022.104711.

Chapter 7

1 Matthew Walker, *Why We Sleep: Unlocking the Power of Sleep and Dreams* (New York: Scribner, 2017).

2 Alicia E. Meuret and Thomas Ritz, "Hyperventilation in Panic Disorder and Asthma: Empirical Evidence and Clinical Strategies," *International Journal of Psychophysiology* 78, no. 1 (2010): 68–79, doi.org/10.1016/j.ijpsycho.2010.05.006.

3 Paul M. Lehrer and Richard Gevirtz, "Heart Rate Variability Biofeedback: How and Why Does It Work?," *Frontiers in Psychology* 5 (2014): art. 756, doi.org/10.3389/fpsyg.2014.00756.

Chapter 8

1 Rachel Kaplan and Stephen Kaplan, *The Experience of Nature: A Psychological Perspective* (Cambridge: Cambridge University Press, 1989); and Stephen Kaplan, "The Restorative Benefits of Nature: Toward an Integrative Framework," *Journal of Environmental Psychology* 15, no. 3 (1995): 169–82, doi.org/10.1016/0272-4944(95)90001-2.

Chapter 9

1 Stephen W. Porges, *The Polyvagal Theory: Neurophysiological Foundations of Emotions, Attachment, Communication, and Self-Regulation* (New York: W. W. Norton, 2011).

Chapter 10

1 Porges, *Polyvagal Theory.*

2 United States Bone and Joint Initiative, *The Impact of Musculoskeletal Disorders on Americans: Opportunities for Action* (Rosemont, IL: United States Bone and Joint Initiative, 2016), based on 2011 data.

3 Ron Z. Goetzel et al., "The Relationship between Modifiable Health Risks and Health Care Expenditures: An Analysis of the Multi-employer HERO Health Risk and Cost Database," *Journal of Occupational and Environmental Medicine* 40, no. 10 (1998): 843–854. See also Ron Z. Goetzel et al., "Ten Modifiable Health Risk Factors Are Linked to More Than One-Fifth of Employer-Employee Health Care Spending," *Health Affairs* 31, no. 11 (2012): 2474–2484.

4 Jonathan Haidt, *The Anxious Generation: How the Great Rewiring of Childhood Is Causing an Epidemic of Mental Illness* (New York: Penguin Press, 2024).

5 *The Social Dilemma*, directed by Jeff Orlowski (2020; Netflix). See also the Center for Humane Technology, cofounded by Tristan Harris.

Chapter 11

1 Francis McGlone, Johan Wessberg, and Håkan Olausson, "Discriminative and Affective Touch: Sensing and Feeling," *Neuron* 82, no. 4 (2014): 737–55, doi.org/10.1016/j.neuron.2014.05.001.

2 James F. Fries, "Aging, Natural Death, and the Compression of Morbidity," *New England Journal of Medicine* 303, no. 3 (1980): 130–35, doi.org/10.1056/NEJM198007173030304.

Chapter 15

1 Elaine Hatfield, John T. Cacioppo, and Richard L. Rapson, *Emotional Contagion* (Cambridge: Cambridge University Press, 1994). On the autonomic transfer specifically, see Richard V. Palumbo et al., "Interpersonal Autonomic Physiology: A Systematic Review of the Literature," *Personality and Social Psychology Review* 21, no. 2 (2017): 99–141.

Index

A

accumulation principle, 23–24, 56, 94–95, 141
acknowledgment, 58
acoustic variety, 41
adaptation, 8, 11, 167
adjustment, 93–95, 184
adolescents, 13, 17, 150. *See also* children
aggregation, 124–125. *See also* accumulation principle
aging, 22–23, 90–91, 141
algorithmic model, 83–85
algorithms
  biometric tracking and, 79–80
  data ownership and, 107
  engagement and, 113
  profit motive and, 109
  scrolling and, 151
  shortcomings of, 87–89
  sympathetic activation and, 151
alignment, 65, 166, 169
allostatic load, 23–24, 94–95
ambient interaction, 106
Android XR, 101
anxiety, 17, 32, 42–43, 59–60, 84
Anxious Generation, The (Haidt), 83
Apollo Neuro, 118
Apple Vision Pro, 100
Apple Watch, 101
artificial intelligence (AI), 96, 102
  coaching, 88, 122, 125
  diagnosis and, 84
  as intelligence, 136
attachment, 27
attentional narrowing, 24–25
attentional recovery, 62–63
attention economy, 108–110
attention regulation, 16
Attention Restoration Theory, 62–63
autonomic nervous system, 15, 32, 55, 88, 90–91, 93, 121
autonomic regulatory development, 16
Ayres, A. Jean, 44

B

Barrett, Lisa Feldman, 34–35
behavior change, problem of, 120
biometrics, 79–80, 101, 117–118
Bolt, Usain, 92
book club, 170–174
Brady, Tom, 92
breathing, 25–26, 31–32, 40, 49–50, 54, 102, 127–128
breath tool kit, 59–60

C
Cacioppo, John, 143
Carney, Dana, 34
Chen, Marcus, 104–105
Chen, Mia, 14–15
children, 13–21, 107, 141. *See also* adolescents
Children's Online Privacy Protection Act, 13
chiropractic, 92–93, 95–96, 146
chronic health conditions, 80–81
ciliary muscles, 40
coaching, 88, 122, 125
cognition, 24–25, 32–34
consistency, 140–141
constructivism, 34–35
cortisol, 41, 55, 90
creativity, 24–25, 33
C-tactile afferent system, 88
Cuddy, Amy, 34

D
data
  giving meaning to, 119–120
  ownership, 107–109
democracy, 151
depression, 17. *See also* anxiety
design
  case, 167
  of heads-up computing, 105–108
  of smartphones, 4–6
development, 16–18, 111–112
dysregulation, 44, 112–113, 152, 180

E
early-adopters, 168–169
embedding, institutional, 144
emotions, 25–26, 34–35. *See also* anxiety
engagement metrics, 106
enthesophytes, 14–15
ergonomics, 63–64
evening, 57–58
expand, in Twenty-Second Lift, 50, 56
eye level, 56, 64, 81, 111, 168

F
faces, 40–41
facial-feedback pathway, 50–51
fascination, 63
Fitbit, 101
freedom, 156–157
Fries, James, 96
future, 152–155

G
Garmin, 101
gaze, 32–34. *See also* eye level
Gevirtz, Richard, 47, 59
Google, 101

H
Haavik, Heidi, 30
Haidt, Jonathan, 83, 108–109
Harris, Tristian, 83, 108–109
Hatfield, Elaine, 143
heads-up computing, 99–116
health, defined, 184
healthcare, defined, 184
health span, 95–97
HeartMath Inner Balance, 118
heart rate, resting, 123
heart rate variability (HRV), 34, 59, 66–68, 84, 102, 118–123, 127–128
hip extension, 57
HRV. *See* heart rate variability (HRV)
Huberman, Andrew, 33
Human Doctor model, 67, 79, 84–98, 128–129, 144, 185

I

information density, 106, 167
Innate Intelligence, 135–137
intelligence, 185. *See also* artificial intelligence (AI); Innate Intelligence; Universal Intelligence
interventions, signals and, 122–125
iPhone, 4–5
Ive, Sir Jony, 5–6

J

Jones, Sophia, 51–53
Jordan, Michael, 92

K

Kaplan, Stephen, 62

L

LaMarche, Gilles, 10, 78, 96–97, 148
lateral movement, 57
leadership, 66, 165–169
Lehrer, Paul, 47
lift, in Twenty-Second Lift, 49
light, natural, 41, 43
Look Up, 121, 128, 185
  in clinical practice, 181–182
  prescribing, 181
  Thirty-Day Look Up Challenge, 163–164

M

Magic Leap, 101
McEwen, Bruce, 23, 94
Meta, 100–103, 110
modeling, 18, 66, 144
monitors, 64
mood, 25–26. *See also* anxiety
morning, 54–56
move, in Twenty-Second Lift, 50
movement, 56–57, 145–146

N

nature, 41–42
nervous system, 118–119, 156–157. *See also* autonomic nervous system; dysregulation; sympathetic activation
neurological development, 16–17, 111–112
Niantic, 101

O

Okafor, James, 25
open, in Twenty-Second Lift, 49
Orion headsets, 100
Oura, 101
outdoors, 41–42
oxytocin, 88, 90

P

pain, defined, 185
pain detector, 83, 177, 185–186
painkiller paradigm, 82–83, 186
PAIN practice, 48–50, 82, 91–95, 113–115, 137–138, 185
partnership, 167–168
pathology detection, 79
patterns, in data, 119–120
Patterson, Keisha, 19–20
performance, 92–93
photoplethysmography (PPG), 102
Porges, Stephen, 72, 151
postural detection, 102, 127
PPG. *See* photoplethysmography (PPG)
presence, 69–73, 144

priority inversion, 136–137
proprioception, 29–31, 46, 48–49, 78, 111–112

Q

Quest headsets, 100
questions, for reading group, 170–174

R

reading group, 170–174
relationships, 26–27, 69–73, 182–183
restraint, 124–125
Reyes, Elena, 71
Ruiz, Daniel, 8–9, 142–143

S

scheduling, state-based, 64–66
Schwarzenegger, Arnold, 92–93
screen-free thresholds, 18
scrolling
  algorithms and, 151
  speed, 113
  sympathetic activation and, 112
self-harm, 17
self-literacy, 125
sensory diet, 39–45, 159, 180–181
60-pound figure, 7
sleep, 57–60, 65, 119, 124, 126–127, 176
smart glasses, 101–105, 110
Snap, 101
social contact, 40–41. *See also* relationships
social vitality synchronization, 128
sounds, 41
Spectacles, 101
spending, healthcare, 80–81, 146–147
spinal extension, 52, 56
spinal rotation, 50, 57, 71
spine
  breathing and, 49–50
  cervical, 4–7, 22–24, 29
  heads-up computing and, 106
  as neural infrastructure, 78–79
  proprioception and, 29–31, 46
state-based scheduling, 64–66
state chain, 35–36
state change, 47–48
stillness, 62–63
suboccipital muscles, 30
suicidal ideation, 13, 17
sympathetic activation, 15–16, 70, 106, 112–113, 123–124, 151
syndrome, 11. *See also* Tech Posture Syndrome

T

technology, 3–4
  benefits of, 114–115
  biometric tracking, 117–118
  categories of, 117–118
  functional support, 118
  leaders, 165–169
  nervous system and, 118–119
  wearable, 101–105
Tech Posture Syndrome, 7, 9–11
  allostatic load and, 23
  children and, 13–21
  presence and, 70–71
  relational cost of, 26–27
Thayer, Julian, 34
thoracic extension, 24
threshold practice, 71–72, 124, 159, 172, 177, 182–183
touch, 41, 43, 87–90
trigger-behavior pair, 51, 182

Tune-In and Tune-Up, 89–91, 94–95, 135–136, 138, 186
tunnel vision mode, 33–34
Twenty-Second Lift, 32, 46–53, 121
  cognitive work and, 33
  Innate Intelligence and, 135–136
  PAIN and, 138
  spine and, 30
  vitality and, 143

U

Universal Intelligence, 133–134

V

vagal state, 70, 72, 113, 151–152
vagus nerve, 31–32
Vaynerchuk, Gary, 113
vision, 32–34
visual breaks, 65
visual system development, 16
vitality, 143–145, 152, 157
Vitality Score, 164
voice interaction, 106
voice stress markers, 124

W

wearables, 101–105
Whoop, 101
workday, 64–66
workforce, 166–167
workplace, 62–68
writing, 33

Z

Zuckerberg, Mark, 110